CHRONIC
NON-CANCER PAIN

This book is dedicated to the millions of people worldwide, whose quality of life is greatly reduced by chronic pain.

CHRONIC NON-CANCER PAIN

ASSESSMENT AND PRACTICAL MANAGEMENT

Edited by

SVEN ANDERSSON
MICHAEL BOND
MARK MEHTA
MARK SWERDLOW

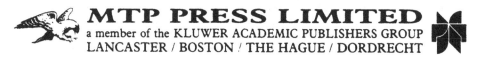

MTP PRESS LIMITED
a member of the KLUWER ACADEMIC PUBLISHERS GROUP
LANCASTER / BOSTON / THE HAGUE / DORDRECHT

Published in the UK and Europe by
MTP Press Limited
Falcon House
Lancaster, England

British Library Cataloguing in Publication Data

Chronic non-cancer pain: assessment and
   practical management.
   1. Pain
   I. Andersson,   Sven
   616'.0472   RB127

   ISBN 0-7462-0046-3
   ISBN 0-7462-0047-1 Pbk

Published in the USA by
MTP Press
A division of Kluwer Academic Publishers
101 Philip Drive
Norwell, MA 02061, USA

Library of Congress Cataloguing in Publication Data

Chronic non-cancer pain.

   Includes bibliographies and index.
   1. Intractable pain. I. Andersson, Sven A. (Sven Anders), 1927–   . [DNLM: 1. Chronic
Disease. 2. Pain—diagnosis. 3. Pain therapy. WL 704 C5565]
RB127.C473 1987   616'.0472   87-13589
ISBN 0-7462-0046-3
ISBN 0-7462-0047-1 (pbk.)

Typeset by Lasertext Ltd., Stretford, Manchester
Printed by Butler and Tanner Ltd., Frome and London

Contents

List of Contributors

Sven Andersson
Professor,
Department of Physiology,
University of Göteborg,
Göteborg,
Sweden

Michael Bond
Professor,
Department of Psychological
  Medicine,
University of Glasgow,
Glasgow,
Scotland

John Bonica
Professor and Former
  Chairman,
Pain Center,
University of Washington,
School of Medicine,
Seattle,
USA

Michael Cousins
Professor and Chairman,
Department of Anaesthesia,
Flinders University of South
  Australia,
Flinders Medical Centre,
Adelaide,
South Australia

Malcolm Jayson
Professor,
Department of Rheumatology,
University of Manchester,
Hope Hospital,
Salford,
Manchester
UK

John Loeser
Department of Neurological
  Surgery,
University of Washington,
School of Medicine,
Seattle,
USA

Mark Mehta
Consultant in Pain Relief,
King Edward VII Hospital,
Midhurst,
Sussex,
UK
(formerly Consultant,
  United Norwich Hospitals)

Ronald Melzack
Professor,
Department of Psychology,
McGill University,
Montreal,
Quebec,
Canada

Harold Merskey
Professor,
Department of Psychiatry,
University of Western Ontario,
London,
Ontario,
Canada

Tim Nash
Consultant,
Department of Anaesthesia,
General Hospital,
Basingstoke,
Hampshire,
UK

William Noordenbos
Professor Emeritus of
  Neurosurgery,
Amsterdam,
Holland

Sydney Rose
Honorary Consultant,
Department of Vascular
  Surgery,
Withington Hospital,
Manchester,
UK

Mark Swerdlow
Honorary Consultant,
N-W Regional Pain Relief
  Centre,
Hope Hospital,
Salford,
Manchester,
UK

Patrick Wall
Professor,
Department of Anatomy, and
  Director, Cerebral Functions
  Research Group,
University College,
London,
UK

Toshikatsu Yokota
Professor,
Department of Physiology,
Medical College of Shiga-Otsu,
Japan

Alistair Young
Consultant,
Department of Neurology,
Hope Hospital,
Salford,
Manchester,
UK

1

Introduction

This book has been written primarily for family doctors and for doctors working in small provincial hospitals who have restricted access to up-to-date medical information. It should also be of interest to medical students and other health care workers.

Our aim has been to provide a clear, uncomplicated but practical account of current practice in the assessment and management of non-cancer pain. For reasons of size and economy we have not attempted to make this volume comprehensive; the emphasis has rather been placed on common conditions and their practical management. We have however included some basic science in order to provide an explanation for the various syndromes and the rationale of treatment. We have throughout recommended only methods which we believe to be safe, practicable and effective. Other methods, which may be more effective but which are more complicated or technically sophisticated, have been mentioned only briefly but reference services for these are provided for interested readers seeking further knowledge.

With regard to drugs we have, on advice, restricted choice to one or two only in each category, being guided by overall effectiveness and cost. Whenever possible selection has been made from the WHO list of essential drugs and genetic names only are employed.

We have been fortunate in enlisting the aid of the experienced and eminent chapter authors who have accepted only token payment of their expenses. A multi-author book poses problems of uniformity of style, presentation and degrees of technicality. We hope that the reader will appreciate our dilemma and not be unduly critical of our editorial decisions.

Those who are inexperienced in pain relief work would be well advised to start at the beginning and read through each section in consecutive order. Those who are seeking answers to specific problems will of course prefer to delve into the appropriate chapters in Parts Three and Four, perhaps referring afterwards to more basic considerations in Parts One and Two.

In most parts of the world much health care is provided by traditional healers. Our introduction of 'Western type' treatment of pain is meant to supplement it or, where appropriate, to provide alternative means of therapy.

The production of this book was supported by the International Association for the Study of Pain (IASP) as a special project in order to provide a wide distribution of basic knowledge in pain therapy to health professionals throughout the world.

Finally we hope that this book will help those practitioners who are far removed from medical libraries and major medical centres and who have no opportunity to attend meetings or join in fruitful discussions with interested colleagues. We also hope that it will do something to improve the quality of life of the many patients worldwide who are in severe chronic pain.

We would be pleased to receive comments and criticism from doctors working in different countries.

ACKNOWLEDGEMENTS

We received useful comments on the original manuscript from a number of workers in several different countries including specialists in different fields, family doctors, medical students and primary health care workers. We are grateful to Prof. J. Thompson, Prof. H. Breivik and to many others who spent a great deal of time to assist us in our task. It is a pleasure to acknowledge the support of Astra Alad A.B., Sweden. Special thanks are also extended to the staff of MTP Press for facilitating the production of this book.

2

Importance of the Problem

John J. Bonica

Introduction

Pain is a complex human experience, the most frequent reason patients seek medical counsel, and the most disabling and costly affliction of mankind. Despite its obvious clinical importance, pain research has been neglected in the past and advances in pain diagnosis and therapy have not been commensurate with most other medical achievements. Fortunately, during the past 15-20 years, a number of developments have taken place which promise to help rectify these deficiencies.

The purpose of this chapter is to emphasize the importance of chronic pain and thus provide a background for the chapters that follow. The material will be presented in three sections: (1) the importance of the problem of chronic pain including its definition and prevalence; (2) an assessment of past and present status of pain therapy and mention of the most important reasons for past deficiencies; (3) brief mention of some of the most important recent and encouraging developments.

Importance of the problem

Today, as in the past, effective therapy for chronic pain remains one of the most pressing issues that should concern society in general, and the medical community in particular. This importance stems from the fact that chronic pain requiring attention from physicians and other health professionals afflicts millions of persons annually, and in many patients it is inadequately relieved by the therapy offered. Consequently pain is the most frequent cause of suffering and disability and seriously impairs the quality of life of millions of people throughout the world daily. In most patients with common disorders such as back ache, arthritis and headache or less common conditions such as facial neuralgia, postherpetic neuralgia, reflex sympathetic dystrophy and many others, pain is the factor that impairs the patient's ability to lead a productive life. Consequently chronic pain is a serious economic problem, as well as a major health problem.

Definition and characteristics of chronic pain

One of the problems that has hampered research, education and health care has been the fact that until recently, it was not recognized that chronic pain is different from acute pain.

Chronic pain is defined as, 'pain that persists beyond the usual course of an acute disease or beyond the reasonable time for an injury to heal'; also it may recur at intervals varying from months to years. Although some clinicians use the arbitrary figure of six months to designate pain as chronic, this is not appropriate because there are many acute diseases or injuries that heal in two, three, or four weeks. Three to four weeks after the condition should have been cured, the pain must be considered chronic. Chronic pain may be caused by chronic pathological processes in somatic structures or viscera, by prolonged dysfunction of parts of the peripheral nervous system or central nervous system, or both. It may also be associated with psychological, sociological and environmental factors.

The mechanisms of persistent chronic pain can be arbitrarily classified as (a) *peripheral mechanisms*, in which the pathology is limited to the tissues or nerve endings; (b) *peripheral-central mechanisms*, in which the initial injury or pathology involves the peripheral nerves that provoke functional changes in the central nervous system that may persist for months and years, as occurs in deafferentation; (c) *central mechanisms*, due to damage of the neuraxis by tumours, surgery, accidental injury, or haemorrhage; and (d) *psychological mechanisms*. It is best to use the term non-malignant chronic pain for chronic pain not associated with cancer.

In addition to the differences mentioned in aetiology and mechanisms, the physiological and psychological effects of chronic pain are much greater and quite different from those of acute pain. Because most of the past research was done on experimentally-induced *acute pain*, our knowledge of the basic mechanisms of chronic pain is meagre. In contrast to acute pain the chronic condition *never* has a biological function, but often imposes severe physical, emotional, economic and social stresses on the patient and the family.

Prevalence and cost of chronic pain

Data suggest that chronic pain syndromes afflict about 30% of the population of industrialized countries. For example, among the 230 million Americans, about 70 million have chronic pain and of these, over 50 million are either partially or totally disabled for periods ranging from a few days (e.g. recurrent headaches) to weeks and months, and some are disabled permanently.

Even more important than the economic impact is the cost in terms of human suffering. It is a distressing fact that in this age of marvellous scientific and technological advances, millions of patients suffer persistent pain that produces serious physical, emotional, and affective disorders. Many patients with chronic pain undergo a progressive physical deterioration caused by disturbance in sleep and appetite, decrease in physical activity, and often excessive medication, all of which contribute to general fatigue and debility.

In addition to anxiety, many patients develop reactive depression, hypochondriasis, somatic preoccupation or a conviction of disease and a tendency to deny life problems unrelated to their physical problem (see Chapter 4).

The social effects of chronic pain are equally devastating; many patients become estranged from their families and friends, decrease their social interactions, and are unable to work and lose their jobs. Some become so discouraged and desperate that they contemplate or even commit suicide.

Status of pain therapy

The many interrelated reasons for deficiencies in pain diagnosis and therapy can be grouped into three major categories: (a) incomplete knowledge about pain and its mechanisms due to insufficient research in the past; (b) inadequate or improper application of available knowledge and therapies; and (c) problems with communication which have resulted in delay in the clinical application of new information about the care of patients with chronic pain.

Recent trends

During the past fifteen years or so, several developments have taken place which, if sustained and expanded, may correct some of the above deficiencies. For example, there has been an impressive surge of interest in the study of chronic pain syndromes and collaboration between basic scientists, clinical investigators and practitioners with a view to solving some of the major clinical problems.

In recent years, there has been better dissemination of information through meetings at national and international levels. This has been reinforced by the publication of monographs and books that contain new and clinically relevant information about pain and its treatment. As a result, the general level of knowledge and interest in pain management has increased steadily.

PART ONE
Basic Mechanisms in Chronic Pain

3

Anatomical, Pathophysiological and Biochemical Aspects of Pain

Sven Andersson and Toshikatsu Yokota

Introduction

Acute pain has an important physiological and protective role as a warning system. A tissue damaging (noxious) stimulus produces an immediate unpleasant sensation together with withdrawal movements and autonomic reflexes. Chronic pain is different; it has no useful physiological purpose. It may result from progressive or sustained tissue damage and it is an outstanding symptom in many diseases. It may also be caused by mechanisms within the nervous system itself without any tissue damage. In chronic pain the emotional state of the patient is important and it may in fact arise from purely psychological disorders. Independent of the cause of the pain the subjective experience and the intensity and quality of the suffering can be judged only by the patient himself. We cannot objectively distinguish the pain after tissue damage from that due to emotions. Therefore, pain can be defined as, 'a sensory and emotional experience associated with actual or potential tissue damage, or described in terms of such damage.' Our knowledge about the mechanisms leading to the sensation of pain is still scanty, particularly concerning the pathophysiology of chronic pain. In the past our knowledge was obtained from

17

the study of acute pain and this was applied to the treatment of chronic pain. The two conditions are entirely different.

CLASSIFICATION

Pain disorders are often classified according to their origin as nociceptive, neurogenic or psychogenic. *Nociceptive* pain arises from stimulation of the nociceptors which are high threshold receptors responding to intense stimulation. The adequate stimulus is tissue damage. Nociceptive pain includes many conditions with inflammatory reaction and tissue destruction. *Neurogenic* chronic pain occurs in conditions where the membrane of the nerve fibres has increased excitability allowing impulse generation in axons in the pain pathways. Such changes can occur at all levels in the pain system, in the afferent peripheral nerve as well as in the central nervous system. The term '*psychogenic pain*' is often used to signify conditions in which no somatic disorder can explain the pain, but where there is evidence of psychological and social precipitating factors. Psychological components are *always* involved in chronic pain as *secondary phenomena*. They may however sometimes be a *primary factor*.

Nociceptive pain

In normal conditions a stimulus gives rise to pain as a result of activity in *nociceptors*. Nociceptors are terminals of myelinated and unmyelinated nerve fibres and they are abundant in the skin as well as in the musculo-skeletal system, for example in fascia, tendon, ligament, joint capsule, periosteum, spongy bone, membranes in the brain and connective tissue in peripheral nerves. On the other hand, there are no nociceptors in the cartilage of joints, the ligamentum flavum, nucleus pulposus of intervertebral discs and compact bone or nervous tissue of the brain and spinal cord.

Most nociceptors in skin, muscles, ligaments and joint capsules respond to different types of tissue damaging stimuli. Some respond only to intense mechanical stimuli, others to mechanical and thermal stimuli and still others, called *polymodal nociceptors*, react to chemical stimuli as well.

The parent afferent fibres of the nociceptors are either thin myelinated A-delta fibres (conduction velocity 10–20 m/s) or slowly conducting unmyelinated C-fibres (conduction velocity 1 m/s). Cutaneous A-delta fibres are characterized by their ability to identify the localisation and intensity of the noxious stimulus and they subserve immediate pricking, cutaneous pain. The C-fibres give rise to the secondary pain which is long lasting, burning and has qualities of aching, suffering and prolonged after-image. The majority of afferent C-fibres are polymodal and have the unique capacity of giving graded responses to mechanical, thermal and chemical stimuli.

Pain arising from deep structures (e.g. ligaments, muscles and joint capsules) has a different character from cutaneous pain. It has a wide distribution and therefore is difficult to localize precisely. Ischaemia is a comon cause of muscle pain. Muscle cells need energy-rich phosphate compounds both during contraction and relaxation. With an adequate supply of oxygen muscle fibres metabolise glycogen which provides sufficient energy but, when there is a lack of oxygen, anaerobic metabolism occurs and the supply of energy is considerably reduced. Consequently ischaemia produces an energy crisis leading to decreased muscle tone and a feeling of stiffness. Potassium ions leak from muscle cells because the Na^+/K^+ pump is no longer fully effective. Local accumulation of extracellular potassium in the exhausted muscle probably increases the excitability of nociceptors. In this situation the sensitivity of the nociceptors increases and normal muscle contractions cause pain.

Chemical mediators of nociceptive pain

If sufficient heat is briefly applied to the skin, burning pain is felt momentarily but it quickly subsides. This pain is probably due to direct physical effects on heat sensitive cutaneous nociceptors. If the heat is just sufficient to scorch the skin visibly, a burning pain develops and lasts for many minutes. The late pain arises from a combination of mechanical and chemical stimulation due to reactions inherent in the inflammatory process with chemical activation of nociceptors by the release of algogenic substances. *Plasma kinins*, such as bradykinin and kallidin, are particularly potent algogenic substances. They are generated from inactive precursors (kininogens) present in the normal plasma and tissues. All of them cause vasodilatation, increased vascular permeability and pain. These effects also make them potential mediators of the inflammatory response. Circulating free plasma kinins are inactivated by kininases found in the blood and tissue.

Serotonin (5–HT) is another powerful algogenic substance which may be released by tissue injury. It is widely distributed in the body, especially in platelets.

Prostaglandins (PGs) are formed by enzymatic oxygenation of unsaturated fatty acids, especially arachidonic acid. Each tissue possesses different synthetic enzymes and therefore produces different types of prostaglandins. When prostaglandins are given in small doses, they do not usually evoke pain. However, PGE_2 (prostaglandin E_2) and prostacyclin (another substance derived from arachidonic acid), in amounts too small to evoke pain alone, cause a state of hyperaesthesia in which the potency of algogenic stimuli is enhanced or in which otherwise minor stimuli become painful. This phenomenon is due to sensitization of the nociceptors. The sensitization of nociceptors by prostaglandins is of considerable importance in the algogenic action of bradykinin. This substance stimulates the biosynthesis of prostaglandins. Both PGE_2 and prostacyclin also produce vasodilatation and potentiate the plasma exudation caused by bradykinin and enhance all aspects of the inflammatory action of bradykinin. Both adrenal glucocorticoids and non-steroidal anti-inflammatory drugs (NSAIDs) like aspirin interfere with the biosynthesis of prostaglandins. The inflammatory reactions induced by bradykinin and derivatives of arachidonic acid are summarized in Figure 1.

Neurogenic pain

Normally sensory nerve fibres transmit impulses which have been generated in specialised receptors. In pathological conditions the

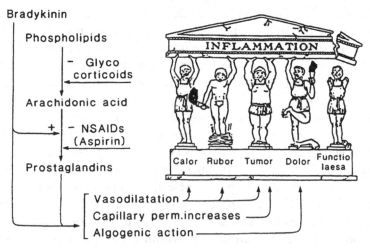

Figure 1 Bradykinin and symptoms of inflammation.

excitability of the nerve fibres themselves increases and impulses are generated in the axonal membrane. The phenomenon is called *ectopic impulse generation*. Nerve damage may also increase the excitability of cells within the central nervous system. Neurogenic pain is often projected pain since it is perceived not at the site where nerve impulses are generated but in the area innervated by the damaged nerve.

Ectopic impulse generation in chronic nerve compression

Normal axons discharge briefly on mechanical distortion as everyone knows who has hit his ulnar nerve at the elbow. Acute nerve compression is dominated by loss of sensitivity and paralysis. If the compression is repeated the excitability of the nerve may increase giving paraesthesia and pain. Post-ischaemic paraesthesia is related to ectopic impulse generation in hyperexcitable nerve fibres. Such discharges are the likely explanation of projected paraesthesia in nerve root pain and in entrapment neuralgia. The mechanism of discharge is related to disturbed membrane mechanisms and is thus different from the sensitization of nociceptors which occurs in inflammatory reactions. These differences between neurogenic and nociceptive pain are reflected in the treatment. Drugs like prostaglandin synthesis inhibitors may relieve nociceptive pain but not neurogenic pain which may be relieved by membrane stabilizing substances like anticonvulsants.

Acute compression of the dorsal root or the dorsal root ganglion produces sustained repetitive discharges. Following rupture of an intervertebral disc, pressure on the nerve root or the dorsal root ganglion may activate nociceptive fibres for many minutes. In long-standing injury dorsal root damage also contributes to the production of continuing radicular pain. Dorsal roots and cutaneous nerves when chronically damaged by pressure show a marked increase in mechanical sensitivity and brief pressure can evoke long-lasting pain.

Pain after nerve transection

The interruption of an axon is followed by Wallerian degeneration of its distal part. During the first week there is also retrograde degeneration in the proximal part for a few millimetres from the cut end. From the cut proximal end of the axon unmyelinated thin nerve sprouts appear. In crush injury severed nerve fibres sprout into a distal Schwann cell tube. The sprouts then reinnervate their proper target cells and other sprouts disappear. If a nerve is transected and its continuity is lost sprouts have no direct pathway to follow; instead they develop into a tissue scar and form a tangled mass called a *neuroma*. A neuroma is a potent source of sharp radiating pain reproduced by tapping over the neuroma. Many thin myelinated and unmyelinated fibres show spontaneous activity. These fibres are sensitive to mechanical stimulation of the neuroma. Their ongoing activity is increased by noradrenaline. Hypersensitivity to noradrenaline partially explains why certain pain conditions, like causalgia, are dependent on noradrenaline release. Such pains can be treated successfully by sympathetic blocking.

Spinal cord mechanisms in pain

As the dorsal root entry zone is approached, primary afferent fibres divide into medial and lateral groups. The thin myelinated A-delta and unmyelinated C-fibres enter the spinal cord via the lateral division of the dorsal root (Figure 4). After entry, they give off ascending branches which run longitudinally for a maximum of two segments in Lissauer's tract and terminate in the grey matter of the dorsal horn.

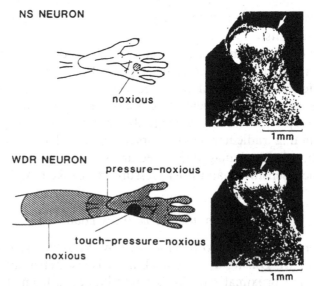

Figure 2 Nociceptive neurons in the spinal dorsal horn. Receptive field and location of a nociceptive specific (NS) neuron are shown in the upper part of the figure, while receptive field and location of a wide dynamic range (WDR) neuron are shown in the lower part of the figure.

Lissauer's tract also contains fibres originating within neighbouring regions of the substantia gelatinosa. Multiple lesions of Lissauer's tract produce a zone of hypalgesia in the related ipsilateral dermatomes, a process which forms the basis of a surgical treatment of chronic pain. Large non-nociceptive afferents enter the spinal cord via the medial division of the dorsal root, and form the large ascending pathway of the dorsal column, but first they give off collaterals to the dorsal horn.

In the *dorsal horn* there are two main classes of nociceptive projection neurons which encode noxious stimulation from the peripheral receptive field. The first type, referred to as *nociceptive specific (NS) neurons*, receive exclusively nociceptive input (Figure 2). They have restricted ipsilateral receptive fields and respond to mechanical stimulation of high intensity. These cells are situated in the most dorsal part of the dorsal horn (lamina I). The second type of nociceptive neurons receive activation from low threshold mechanical stimulation in addition to input from ipsilateral nociceptors. As a result they are sometimes called *wide dynamic range* (WDR) cells. Such cells are located in lamina I and lamina V of the dorsal horn. They respond to brush, touch, pressure and noxious mechanical stimulation in the centre of the receptive field, but only to intense mechanical stimulation in the periphery of the field (Figure 2). The neurons receiving input from noxious stimulation in the dorsal horn transmit activity through a pathway which crosses the midline and reaches the ventrolateral part of the spinal cord. It then ascends in the spinothalamic tract.

The organisation of the input to the pain pathway from the skin is different from that of the input from deep tissue (myotome, sclerotome). Deep pain is often referred to other deep structures with the same segmental innervation; a characteristic feature which does not occur after stimulation of cutaneous nociceptors. For example, pain in the hip joint frequently gives pain in the region of the greater trochanter and also at the anterior side of the thigh. The explanation is that the innervation of the hip joint (acetabulum and femoral head) reaches the same segment as the skeletal and muscle afferents from these regions. The convergence of nerve fibres from different deep structures is similar to the convergence from visceral and somatic afferents. In general, pain from deep structures is less well localized than cutaneous pain. Deep pain is also different in quality and is described as aching without the burning and sharp components characteristic of cutaneous pain.

Spinal reflexes in pain

The nociceptive afferents have synaptic connections with motor neurons and with sympathetic efferent neurons in the spinal cord. In acute pain the reflex via flexor motoneurons causes withdrawal. At the same time sympathetic neurons mediate accompanying vasomotor and respiratory changes (Figure 3). These reflexes are important also in chronic pain because they may cause sustained muscle contractions and ischaemia.

Nociceptive impulses generated by painful tissue damage cause reflex muscle contraction to protect injured areas of the body. The ongoing afferent discharges give a tonic muscle contraction. The muscle activity stimulates muscle nociceptors and nerve impulses are fed back to the central nervous system. In certain conditions nociceptive impulses may converge on the motoneurons producing muscle contraction (Figure 3A). A vicious circle is formed and muscle contraction is sustained producing a pain more severe than that of

A   Motor vicious circle

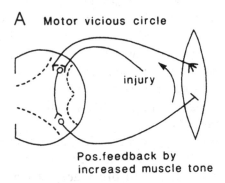

Pos.feedback by
increased muscle tone

B   Autonomic vicious circle

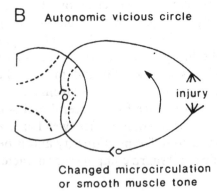

Changed microcirculation
or smooth muscle tone

Figure 3   Motor (A) and sympathetic (B) reflex couplings underlying chronic pain.

the original injury. A similar phenomenon can occur in the sympathetic system (Figure 3B) as in cardiac ischaemia. Nociceptors are activated due to inadequate oxygen supply which results in an increased sympathetic tone.

The involvement of sympathetic vasoconstriction is important also in the tonic (skeletal muscle) contraction following tissue damage. During muscle exercise and energy crises (see p.19) there is marked vasoconstriction causing a decrease in the blood supply to the muscle. The result will be further pain, decreased muscle power and stiffness. The sustained pain in such a situation can be related to increased discharges in both muscle and sympathetic efferents. This is exemplified by primary fibromyalgia which is characterized by pain, muscle weakness and stiffness. Trigger points are often located in the trapezius and brachioradialis muscles. Biopsies taken from these muscles in a patient with fibromyalgia show low and uneven oxygen tension and a low content of energy-rich phosphate compounds.

The transmission of impulses through the synapses in the somatic and sympathetic nociceptive reflexes is influenced by segmental and suprasegmental control. An important role is played by the 'gate control' mechanism described by Melzack and Wall. As indicated in Figure 4 the large diameter fibres transmitting information from low threshold afferents such as touch, pressure and vibration have an inhibitory effect on transmission in the pain pathways. Impulses in these fibres act as a brake on the passage of activity in the nociceptive

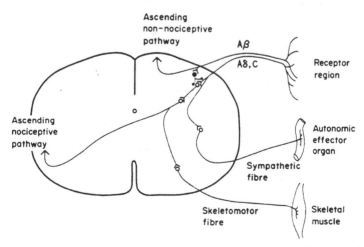

Figure 4 Schematic drawing of connections from nociceptive and non-nociceptive afferents in the spinal cord.

pathway.

The inhibitory influence on the nociceptive pathway can be artificially increased by activating myelinated fibres. Touch, pressure or vibration decrease the response of cells in the dorsal horn to nociceptive stimulation. Pain sensation and the reflex responses are also diminished. Transcutaneous electrical nerve stimulation (TENS) which is used to relieve pain is based on segmental inhibition of the pain pathway.

Visceral and referred pain

Impulses which evoke visceral pain arrive in the central nervous system via myelinated A-delta and unmyelinated C-fibres. In the digestive system nociception is mostly mediated via the splanchnic nerves. Certain forms of gastrointestinal discomfort associated with ulcers apparently originate from activity in the vagal afferents. Pain originating from the heart is due to activity in the sympathetic cardiac afferents. Pain originating from the respiratory and pelvic organs is largely initiated by afferent fibres which travel with the parasympathetic nerves. In the visceral organs, there are several specialized sensory receptors that must be recognized as nociceptors.

Pain arising from the visceral organs is generally diffuse and difficult to localize. It is often referred to the somatic segments supplied by the dorsal roots through which the visceral afferent impulses reach the spinal cord. The pain of angina pectoris may be localized exclusively to its site of origin behind the sternum, but frequently it tends to radiate to the left shoulder, thence down the left arm to the elbow or to the wrist. Sometimes, the pain starts in the left wrist, arm or shoulder and radiates towards the sternum. Detailed consideration of the physiology of visceral pain is more appropriately considered together with the clinical features. The reader is referred to Chapter 10.

Trigeminal mechanisms

Many trigeminal nerve fibres bifurcate in the pons. One branch proceeds to the trigeminal main sensory nucleus, and another branch joins the descending spinal tract of the trigeminal nerve. The descending spinal tract projects to the spinal tract nucleus of the trigeminal nerve. Surgical section of the descending spinal tract (trigeminal tractotomy) at the level of the obex eliminates trigeminal pain and thermal sensations at the side of the lesion. This operation interrupts trigeminal input to the subnucleus caudalis which is the rostral continuation of the dorsal horn of the cervical cord.

Ascending pathways of nociception

Lesions of the anterolateral part of the spinal cord can cause complete contralateral loss of pain and temperature sensitivity with intact sensation to touch on both sides. The nerve fibres conducting temperature and pain decussate and the information is conducted in ventrolateral spinothalamic pathways on the opposite side. Patients with bilateral ventrolateral lesions of the spinal cord will be numb below the level of the lesion. Tactile sensation is conducted by the posterior columns on the same side, and this path decussates after its synapse in the dorsal column nuclei.

Anterolateral cordotomy is an accepted treatment for intractable pain. This procedure divides the anterolateral spinothalamic tract and also ascending pathways transmitting other sensations such as touch and pressure. Pain relief is not permanent; after a varying period of time pain returns sometimes accompanied by dysaesthesia. For this reason the procedure is not recommended for the patient with a long life expectancy.

Thalamic mechanisms of nociception

The ascending nociceptive pathways terminate in several thalamic nuclei which in turn project to different areas of the cerebral cortex. Some aspects of pain sensation, such as its location and quality, are relayed via the thalamic nuclei where somatic sensations like touch and pressure are represented. The unpleasant, aversive aspects of the pain sensation are mediated via other thalamic regions. At both the thalamic and cortical levels there is interaction between the pain pathways and other somatic pathways. A mechanism similar to the gate control in the spinal cord operates at this level. Central pain which can arise after lesions in the thalamus may be due to removal of inhibitory influence.

Cortical mechanisms of pain

It is thought that pain and temperature sensation are represented in the front part of the postcentral gyrus. There are patients with focal parietal lobe lesions in whom pain and other sensibility are grossly impaired on the contralateral side of the body. Damage to the posterior bank of the central sulcus causes loss of pain, temperature, and touch sensations as well as the ability to discriminate. In contrast patients with lesions in the lateral aspects of the postcentral gyrus suffer permanent loss of discriminatory ability only. Electrical stimulation of the postcentral gyrus in conscious subjects commonly elicits sensations such as numbness and tingling on the contralateral side, but rarely pain.

The nature of the pain is further elucidated in the inferior lobule of the posterior parietal cortex. Lesions in this part of the cortex of the dominant hemisphere may produce an asymbolia for pain in which the patient is unable to recognize the unpleasant or disagreeable components of a painful stimulus, although the noxious stimulus itself is perceived.

Inhibitory pathways of nociception

Inhibitory mechanisms in the descending pathways from the brainstem together with those in the spinal cord play an important role in the central integration of nociception. Electrical stimulation of brainstem sites produces profound suppression of the response to noxious stimuli. Important structures in this respect are located in periventricular grey which surrounds the third ventricle, the mesencephalic periaqueductal grey, nucleus raphe magnus and its adjacent nucleus reticularis magno-cellularis in the medulla oblongata. From these nuclei pathways descend in the dorsolateral funiculus of the spinal cord (Figure 5). Particularly in nucleus raphe magnus there are serotoninergic (5-HT) neurons with axons reaching to the dorsal horn where they exert inhibition on nociception. There are similar mechanisms in the trigeminal subnucleus caudalis.

There are several descending systems which inhibit nociception. Some of them operate via endogenous opioid peptides. They affect the reaction to pain rather than the specific perception of pain. They do not markedly influence other sensory modalities such as touch, vision and hearing. This rather unusual specificity of morphine and the opioid peptides is due to interaction with specific receptors referred to as *opioid receptors*. They are widely distributed throughout the central nervous system with high density in particular regions like the superficial layers of the dorsal horn and the trigeminal subnucleus caudalis. Internally produced opioids exert a strong pain-relieving

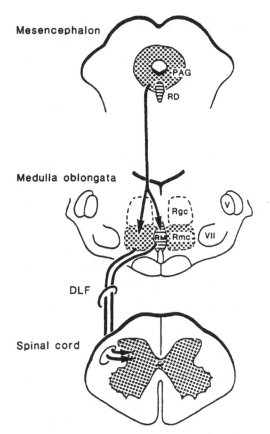

Figure 5 Descending inhibitory pathway of nociception. PAG: periaqueductal grey matter. RD: nucleus raphe dorsalis. Rgc: nucleus reticularis gigantocellularis. RM: nucleus raphe magnus. Rmc: nucleus reticularis magnocellularis.

effect by attachment to specific receptors in the nervous system.

Prominent among the endogenous opioids are the pentapeptides methionine-enkephalin (met-enkephalin) and leucine-enkephalin (leu-enkephalin). Corticotrophin-beta-lipotrophin precursor is produced by corticotroph cells in the pituitary and the basal hypothalamus. This protein is the common precursor of corticotrophin (ACTH) and beta-endorphin; a potent analgesic slowly inactivated by enzymes. Met-enkephalin and leu-enkephalin are also found in the brain and spinal cord. They have a weak analgesic action and are rapidly inactivated by aminopeptidases. Beta-neoendorphin, dynorphin, leu-morphine and rimorphin are found in the hypothalamus and other brain structures as well as in the spinal cord.

Noradrenaline and serotonin modulate the nociceptive process in the dorsal horn. Interference with serotonin neurons by pharmacological blockade reduces the effectiveness of systemic opioids, suggesting that endorphinergic and serotoninergic pathways are linked together. On the other hand, anti-depressant drugs which block 5-HT reuptake and reinforce 5-HT transmission give pain relief and potentiate opioid analgesia. The use of anti-depressive drugs in clinical pain is therefore directed towards both the 'psychic' components and the inhibition of the nociceptive message.

The powerful analgesic effect of the spinal inhibition of nociception is clearly demonstrated by intrathecal administration of morphine. The effect is presumably due to diffusion of the drug into the dorsal horn with binding to opioid receptors which activates inhibitory mechanisms.

Endorphinergic systems in the midbrain and spinal cord are not fully understood. They operate as a negative feed-back loop in response to pain or stress. These mechanisms may be involved in acupuncture, transcutaneous electrical nerve stimulation (TENS) and related therapies. High frequency stimulation activates non-opioid mechanisms, whereas low frequency stimulation at higher intensity induces analgesia via opioid activity. There is clear evidence that prolonged activation is necessary and 10–20 minutes stimulation is often required to give the best pain relief. Pain modulation frequently outlasts the period of stimulation. It should be pointed out that these stimulation techniques require an intact midbrain and spinal cord.

Recommended reading

1. Wall, P.D. and Melzack, R. (1984). *Textbook of Pain.* (Edinburgh: Churchill Livingstone) (Comprehensive but expensive, suitable for libraries)
2. Willis, W.P. (1985). *The Pain System.* (Basel: Karger)

4

Psychology of Pain

Michael Bond

Introduction

Pain is a personal experience and a symptom of disease or injury, but not a disease in itself. Irrespective of its cause or severity, experience of pain involves changes in both emotion and behaviour, the details of which will be discussed later in this chapter.

Pain usually arises as a result of physical disease or injury and the previous chapter described the routes taken by noxious impulses through the nervous system. In particular it is known that the more slowly conducting pathways deliver impulses over a wide area in the brain, including those responsible for the generation and control of emotional events and associated changes in behaviour.

In addition to physically induced pain there is a small proportion of patients with disorders for which no causative disease or injury is known. Analysis of peripheral nerve activity and events in the spinal cord fail to reveal any abnormality but, nevertheless, the sufferer complains of pain. We are now fully aware that pain may develop in certain emotional disorders and, in fact, complaints of pain are common amongst patients attending doctors for the treatment of these disorders. Often such pain has its own characteristics; it bears no relation to any known regional or dermatome pattern associated with tissue damage, nor is it necessarily of the same quality as pain arising from a specific organic disorder. However, there are times when the pain occurs at the site of a previous injury or surgical lesion, and this may cause considerable difficulties with diagnosis.

These general comments make it clear that understanding the nature of emotions in relation to pain is essential to both the analysis of a person's pain problem and to its treatment irrespective of its origins.

Culture and pain

Cultural attitudes to pain and suffering exert a very powerful influence over the behaviour of pain sufferers and the use of pain complaints as symbols of emotional distress or social difficulties of certain types. Perhaps the most obvious effect of culture upon pain is the way in which it influences *complaint behaviour*. In broad terms each culture has its own patterns of complaint behaviour amongst the sick and injured. In some countries, it is regarded as important not to complain excessively about physical symptoms – especially pain – and this view is particularly strong amongst men. As the general attitude is shared by both doctors and patients, it means that pain is often very poorly treated in even the most technically sophisticated hospitals and medical institutes. In other societies, there is freedom to complain about pain and some evidence that this brings both personal relief to the sufferer and mobilisation of sympathy and attention from family, friends and those caring for the sick. In brief, there are great variations in attitudes to suffering and pain and with them certain differences in approaches to pain control.

The presentation of emotional problems as physical complaints, appears to be a universal phenomenon. There are many individuals from a wide variety of educational and social backgrounds who have pain for which psychosocial rather than biological causes can be found. In some societies pain is totally symbolic of certain socially well recognised problems. For example, in one North African culture a father's complaint of pain in his knee may symbolise displeasure or disappointment with a favourite son. In this case pain is playing a part in a complex social ritual which involves suffering but not that brought about by a physical event. Similar processes, though perhaps not so immediately obvious, exist in Western society also. Thus, facial pain without an obvious cause is in some cases symbolic because it represents the inability of the sufferer 'to face' a significant person in his life with whom he is experiencing considerable emotional difficulties which are not openly discussed, but which generate a very obvious and powerful state of tension between the two individuals.

Personality and pain

An individual's personality is his or her 'mental signature tune' and consists of those complex qualities of intellect, emotions and behaviour which differ from one person to another in such a way as to make almost all of us unique. Perhaps only in the case of identical twins do we find identical, or almost identical, personality characteristics. Despite the subtle differences that exist between us however, there are readily identifiable common qualities which are possessed by most people and although they are greatly influenced by factors such as age and cultural origin, they are qualities found in all mankind.

Perhaps an individual's tendency to become anxious or feel depressed is the most basic human emotion which influences pain. In simple terms the greater the ease with which a person feels anxious, and is anxious when in pain, the greater will be the level of pain experienced. In acute pain anxiety is the over-riding emotion and its control is of major importance. In contrast, chronic pain sufferers have feelings of misery, loss of hope, loss of self-esteem and social loneliness which give rise to depression. In such cases much of the suffering and pain can be reduced by practical help, advice and counselling, without resorting to the use of powerful analgesic or psychotropic drugs. Mention of pain sensitivity is appropriate at this point and there are two levels of measurement. '*Pain perception threshold*' is the point at which an increasing stimulus becomes painful and this varies very little from one person to another. Increasing the stimulus produces increasing pain; the point at which this becomes unbearable is the '*tolerance level*' which varies widely between people and even with each person from time to time. The difference between these two is a measure of an individual's range of pain tolerance. The tolerance level is reduced by anxiety and depression and may be increased by cultural attitudes, sporting activities and, paradoxically, by states of overwhelming anxiety and aggression as, for example, in battle or physical combat.

In addition to anxiousness and depressiveness, the personality traits bear a relationship to pain experience and behaviour. In order of importance they are hypochondriasis, hysterical characteristics, and tendencies towards obsessional behaviour.

Hypochondriasis

The development of specific attitudes to health and sickness occurs in all people in all societies and must of course be influenced by cultural factors. Nevertheless, a tendency to be concerned about health and changes in the body is probably universal and a normal human condition. The tendency to be excessively concerned, or hypochondriacal, becomes a problem when it gives rise to anxiety about the body amounting to a fear and perhaps belief that a physical disorder exists. Some individuals are lifelong hypochondriacs but others only develop hypochondriacal fears when under stress of an emotional or social kind and this pattern should be looked for when the possibility of hypochondriasis is being considered. The hypochondriacal trait frequently results in self-medication (often with analgesics and sometimes to a dangerous degree) and also to excessive dependence on doctors. The dangers for the hypochondriacal person in such a system are of over-investigation and over-treatment. Pain is a frequent symptom amongst the hypochondriacal and may arise in any part of the body; there may well be a physical basis for it but often this is trivial. Also there is a tendency for patients to experience multiple symptoms together or in sequence and therefore complaints may be of different kinds and in different areas of the body at different times. Finally a doctor's awareness that a patient is hypochrondriacal has another potential danger – that of missing symptoms and signs of a major physical problem after repeated requests for treatment for trivial conditions.

Hysterical traits

Individuals with an histrionic personality show immaturity in their emotions and behaviour. They exhibit a constant need to be the centre of attention, they form rather shallow emotional relationships with others, tend to exaggerate their experiences in life whether pleasant or unpleasant, and when ill, become excessively demanding of others' time and attention. In addition, individuals with marked hysterical traits tolerate poorly the symptoms of physical disease or injury. Often this will bring them in contact with a doctor or with other medical professionals who are unable to meet the individual's demands for personal attention and rapid relief of pain with the result that tensions may lead to a breaking of the patient's relationship with medical or other staff.

Obsessional traits

The individual with marked obsessional characteristics is not uncommon, particularly amongst professional groups where orderliness, punctuality, reliability, a high moral tone and an ability to adhere to strict routines have some advantages. However, the need for orderliness and abhorrence of uncertainty may make the diagnosis and treatment of painful physical illness an ordeal for both doctor and patient. The doctor is often asked for excessive amounts of information about causes and treatments that will produce symptom relief without the side effects and the patient, driven by uncertainty, may well develop high levels of emotional tension and find difficulty in coping with the physical and emotional consequences of ill health. The doctor is most likely to cope with such a patient if he is truthful and as concise in his opinion as possible, giving good reasons for any inability to answer questions completely. Such a course will reduce the sufferer's degree of uncertainty to a bearable level and reduce tension leading to an increased tolerance for symptoms, including pain.

Learned behaviour and pain

Clearly there are great individual variations in the way in which people perceive illness in themselves and others, the emotional responses they display and the behaviour they exhibit. In fact, much of what we feel and do is 'learned behaviour' which develops as a result of contact with close relatives and peers during our childhood years.

It is important to realise that illness or injury alter an individual's social health status and, for a time, he or she occupies what is known as the 'sickness role'. Whilst in the sickness role, each of us behaves in a certain way and this is known as 'sickness behaviour', and an understanding of this concept is essential for satisfactory analysis of pain problems. Finally, the term 'somatisation' is used to describe the process by which an individual's emotional and/or social distress is presented to a doctor as a physical symptom. The patient may be aware of the process but more often seems totally unaware that his symptoms have their origins in emotional or social problems.

The sickness role and sickness behaviour

In all societies an ill person takes up what is called 'the sickness role'. This is a state granted to the individual by society which expects him or her to report illness as unacceptable, and in which he is expected to make every effort to collaborate with doctors, medical personnel or traditional healers. In addition, the sick are expected to use all resources available to them in order to get well as quickly as possible. In most cases an individual in the sick role is freed from the usual responsibilities of life at home and at work for as long as there seems to be a genuine physical basis for the illness. Therefore, as in the case of health, illness is a well recognised state and carries with it certain accepted forms of behaviour and even certain duties. For instance, with regard to behaviour, a person may be very stoical when ill and in pain, or in contrast, may behave histrionically or emotionally. It is clear that behaviour includes both what a person says about his symptoms and non-verbal movements and gestures. In some cases, both words and actions match in the way we expect – for example, when a patient with renal colic describes agonising pain, is pale, sweating and has facial distortion whilst at the same time clasps the hand over the affected area. In certain disorders patients' words may *not* match their behaviour and such a discrepancy is important in the recognition of pains attributable more to psychological and social rather than physical causes.

A small proportion of people find that illness gives them protection against unwelcome stresses produced by the responsibilities of everyday life. Such protection is rewarding and therefore the individual tends to prolong his occupancy of the sick role and is said to show 'abnormal sickness behaviour'. Some individuals develop this style of behaviour as a consequence of disease or injury during childhood when abnormal sickness behaviour is common, though generally brief. Others do not do so until they encounter a serious illness in adult life when they learn that their unmet needs for affection, protection, or dependency can be fulfilled by maintenance of their symptoms and where abnormal sickness behaviour is reinforced by full or partial satisfaction of such needs. From the reader's point of view, what constitutes normal and abnormal sickness behaviour will be particular to his own society and culture.

What has been written so far refers to changes in feelings, attitudes and behaviour amongst individuals who are afflicted by disease or injury of a physical nature. Thus small numbers of people move into 'abnormal sickness behaviour' for various reasons. In addition, there are others who develop signs and symptoms suggesting painful disease or injury without evidence of an organic basis for their symptoms. The process involved is known as 'somatisation'.

Somatoform disorders

The essential features of a somatoform disorder are:

'physical symptoms suggesting a physical disorder for which there are no demonstrable findings or known physiological mechanisms and for which there is positive evidence or a strong presumption that the symptoms are linked to psychological factors or conflicts'.

It is important to note that the symptoms are *not* under voluntary control which means that the sufferer does not feel that he or she has control over them. The individual who has a somatisation disorder presents with recurrent somatic complaints, often over many years. He receives a good deal of medical attention in most cases but a physical cause is not detected. The patient may present with pain alone or with multiple somatic symptoms including pain. Although complaints of mild tension and depression are frequent amongst such patients, a primary diagnosis of mental illness should not be made (see page 39).

Somatisation disorder

The disorder of somatisation often begins in adolescence or early adult life. Headache, abdominal or other pains, feelings of depression and many other possible physical symptoms (Table 1) are presented

Table 1 Diagnostic criteria for a somatisation disorder

1. A history of physical symptoms of several years duration beginning in adolescence or early adult life.
2. Multiple complaints (at least 14 for women and 12 for men) from the areas listed below. The complaints must have been sufficient to interrupt the patient's way of life significantly, have led to consultations with doctors, and treatments other than very simple domestic remedies. There should not be evidence of physical disease or injury sufficient to explain the symptoms.

    Symptom Groups
    (a) Non-specific lifelong ill health.
    (b) Gastro-intestinal symptoms – including abdominal pain.
    (c) Cardiopulmonary symptoms – including chest pain.
    (d) Neurological or pseudoneurological symptoms.
    (e) Urogenital symptoms in the female reproductive tract – including pelvic pain.
    (f) Psychosexual symptoms – including pain during intercourse.
    (g) Complaints of pain – for example, in the back, joints, extremities, genital area (other than during intercourse) pain on urination and other pains, excluding headaches.

over a period of time and *the course of the disorder is chronic and fluctuating*. Studies of such patients show that seldom does a year pass without some form of medical attention. A long history of medical assessments and often of unnecessary investigations and treatment will be found where such facilities are available. Despite constantly or nearly constantly being in the sick role, the patient's family often seem to adjust to this situation and indeed attempts to restore more normal behaviour are often not only unsuccessful but resisted by patients and family members alike. Moreover, any attempt to break up the family's patterns of behaviour may lead to an emotional crisis involving several family members.

Table 1 gives the diagnostic criteria for a somatisation disorder.

Psychogenic pain disorder

A number of patients present with the *single* complaint of pain for which *no* organic cause can be found. The pain may occur anywhere in the body but is most frequent in the face or head, back or abdomen. The distribution and nature of the pain are not characteristic of known physical disorders but have the characteristics of pain brought about by psychological factors. It is commonly described as being present throughout the day but does not wake the patient from sleep, and it does not respond, other than briefly, to conventional medicines or physical treatments for pain relief. As in the case of the somatisation disorder, pain has often been present for many years and the patient will have undergone many investigations and treatments. In some patients evidence of secondary muscle spasm may be found and there may even be parasthesiae in the limbs. The diagnostic criteria for

Table 2   Diagnostic criteria for a psychogenic pain disorder

1. Severe prolonged pain (usually present for several years).

2. Pain inconsistent with the anatomic distribution of the nervous system and for which no organic, pathological or pathophysiological mechanism can be found. When related or organic pathology is present, the complaint of pain is grossly in excess of what would be expected.

3. Psychological factors are to be regarded as aetiologically important if one or more of the following criteria is fulfilled:

    (a) A temporal relationship between pain and the presence of a psychological conflict or need.

    (b) The fact that pain enables an individual to avoid unwanted or unpleasant activities.

    (c) Pain which leads to some form of gain that would not be forthcoming in its absence.

4. There should be no evidence of other mental disorder.

psychogenic pain disorder are given in Table 2.

Table 3 shows how to determine the extent to which physical and psychological elements contribute to pain states.

Mental illness and pain

Patients with psychiatric disorders are known to experience pain and, in fact, about half of all patients attending psychiatric clinics include pain amongst their symptoms. Three groups of disorders are considered.

1. Neuroses with pain.

2. Psychosomatic disorders.

3. Major mental illness and pain.

Table 3   Indications of physical and psychological elements in pain states

Indications of marked physical elements in a pain state	Indications of marked psychological and behavioural elements in a pain state
Onset. Usually clearcut.	Vague or uncertain. Often no precipitating factor.
Nature. Well recognized characteristics, e.g. colic, pain of myocardial infarction etc. Interferes with sleep.	Often not well described. May be a discrepancy between severity described and behaviour. Often not present during night hours.
Site. Usually recognized by its relation to injury or disease or to its site if referred.	Ill-defined in some cases. In others may occur at site of previous tissue damage (trauma, surgery, etc.) More often on left side of body.
Increased by movement, palpation etc.	Increased by wide range of stimuli, or unchanged by any stimulus. May change in relation to mood variation.
Relieved by physical means, i.e. rest, analgesics, surgery, etc.	Anxiolytic drugs, alcohol and other methods of reducing emotional tension. Often said to be unresponsive to any treatment.
Other features. Psychological factors prominent as secondary changes, i.e. development of depression or anxiety.	Commonly premorbid history of neurotic traits or mental illness. The latter are usually neurotic disorders.

Neuroses with pain

The neuroses most commonly associated with pain are anxiety and depressive neuroses. Hypochondriasis described previously is a common feature of both conditions referring to the fear patients have that their symptoms, however slight, signify serious illness or injury. Hysterical characteristics modify the way in which patients present their symptoms.

Anxiety neurosis and pain

Anxiety neurosis is a state in which excessive anxiety occurs amounting to acute fear or even panic at times. Somatic symptoms also develop due to alterations in the activity of the autonomic nervous system and to a lesser extent of the endocrine system. The changes in an individual's emotional and physical state have secondary effects upon his intellectual activities, including impairment of concentration and memory and judgement. Anxiety reactions are common but vary in form, some patients complaining chiefly of emotional tension, whereas others are concerned primarily with physical symptoms. The former describe feelings of being 'tense', 'strung up' or 'on edge', all expressions which give the sensation of tension. Complaints of excessive anxiety, constant nervousness and of being in a panic are common, and those who have experienced tachycardia, excessive sweating, dryness of the mouth and trembling may interpret their physical feelings in more general terms, such as having trembling of the stomach or shortness of breath which at times amounts to choking. They may feel that they are about to collapse or even die. The anxious person is restless, unable to sit still for any length of time and, in less acute conditions, tends to complain of tiredness, loss of energy and insomnia. Their eating habits change and there may be either increased or decreased appetite. Usually there are difficulties in sleep, with initial sleeplessness and later restlessness and sudden frequent awakening.

Amongst those with chronic anxiety most complaints are related to the head and neck, back or abdomen, and chest in that order of frequency. Headaches are often described as a 'tight band' or a 'weight on the head', and the feeling of tension and pain may extend down into the neck or even further into the large paravertebral muscles of the back. Palpation of large muscle groups, for example in the lumbar and cervical region, shows that they are tender to the touch and that movement of that part of the body is not only limited but associated with increased pain. In some areas 'trigger points' may be found. They are exquisitely tender regions beneath which nodules can be felt in the muscle. When pressed, these give rise to local acute pain which is often referred to more distant parts of the body. The symptoms constitute the basis of what is often known as the *myofascial syndrome*. Usually the patient's history and emotional state are sufficient to explain the presence of pain in muscles; however, the diagnosis of a tension state should not be accepted as the basis for pain until a reasonable search for organic sources has been made.

Reactive depression and pain

Depression occurs quite commonly in response to identifiable stresses in the environment (for example the death of a close relative) and when it does so the sufferer retains contact with the reality of the surrounding world and is not troubled by delusions or hallucinations. This form of depression is regarded as *reactive* or neurotic. It is different from severe depressive illness with psychotic features and from manic depressive psychosis. A depressive neurosis is expressed by changes of mood, intellect and physical health. Depressed people feel miserable and this is aggravated by thinking of the factors giving rise to depression. It tends to be worse when the individual is alone and less severe when he is in the company of others or situations which distract the mind. There is a sense of loss, of joy having gone out of life and there are associated feelings of hopelessness and pessimism about the future. The levels of energy and interest fall, concentration, memory and judgement deteriorate, and physical symptoms of various kinds may appear. It is common for patients to experience a change in appetite, sometimes with overeating and a marked increase in weight, and sometimes with almost total loss of appetite and marked weight loss. Sleep is impaired and the night is troubled by dreams with a depressive content and periods of wakefulness. Complaints of aches and pains are common in depressive disorders which are a reaction to obvious stresses in life and are also associated with a tendency to develop hypochondriasis as part of physical illness.

Pain and psychosomatic disorders

It is clear that every form of illness has emotional aspects and social consequences but, in certain instances, the disease process appears to be initiated or prolonged by disturbances of emotional life and/or by adverse social factors. Those illnesses in which this mechanism appears to be particularly active are known as 'Psychosomatic Disorders'. Familiar and common examples of the conditions in which major physiological changes occur in response to stress include asthma, peptic ulceration, migraine, ulcerative colitis and the irritable bowel syndrome. Some of these include pain amongst their symptoms. It has been shown that those who suffer from psychosomatic disorders exhibit certain characteristics including the strong possibility of the same type of illness occurring in relatives or a personal history of more than one psychosomatic disorder. Psychosomatic disorders tend to be intermittent, appearing in times of stress whether purely emotional, environmental or some combination of the two. Psychosomatic disorders appear to be specific to each individual and the members of the families who suffer them. In other words, the development of migraine, for example, is one person's way of responding to emotional stress and strain whereas another person develops symptoms of peptic ulcer and a third of ulcerative colitis. This way of responding to the pressures of life is generally understood by the sufferer and the doctor as both are able to link cause and effect without difficulty and to establish a relationship for the treatment of physical symptoms which not only sustains the patient but perhaps also leads to a discussion and relief of the stressful factors causing them. Therefore, for the most part painful psychosomatic disorders are dealt with very adequately on a physical basis but experience shows that their psychological management often leaves much to be desired, given that many doctors are far more comfortable with the use of physical treatments rather than with dealing with emotional disturbances.

Major mental illness and pain

A psychotic depressive disorder differs from reactive depression in that there is less often an obvious precipitating factor, the level of depression is more constant, and is not affected by changes of circumstances. It tends to be more pronounced in the early part of the day. Often it is associated with delusions which are firmly held but false, such as beliefs that the individual is doomed or that he is poor, or has been the cause of distress to others. In some cases depression is associated with restlessness or agitation; in others with apathy which may lead to complete immobility or depressive stupor. In psychotic depression, appetite is lost and there may be very rapid reduction of weight. There is also loss of sexual interest and the individual's depression may reach such a depth that he contemplates suicide. Pain is not a common complaint in patients with severe psychotic depression but when it occurs it may be a prominent symptom even to the extent of overshadowing the depression. Fears of serious physical illness may be present also; for example, the patient may believe that he has cancer or venereal disease.

The treatment of depression by conventional methods, chiefly the use of antidepressant drugs, will relieve both depression and pain.

Malingering

The differentiation of true diseases from malingering is one of the difficulties of clinical life. However, there are several clues which should give rise to a suspicion of malingering – a state in which an individual consciously and deliberately falsifies physical symptoms including pain. In Western countries the motive is most often monetary gain as compensation for some form of alleged injury at work or in an accident. Clinical examination may reveal a physical abnormality but it will either be very slight in comparison with the level of disability, or obviously be manufactured. Pain is an ideal symptom for a malingerer because it is difficult to measure, disprove and investigate. Careful observation of the patient, however, may reveal that behaviour is normal when he believes he is alone. Further investigation may uncover a previous history of similar events of dishonesty or of family problems, especially financial ones, for which some dramatic solution is required. Although the patient will not be at work often, he has not given up his pleasures in life. It is possible that he will not submit to hospitalisation, surgery or major investigation and may default on any treatment given. Offers of employment are often refused even though they may involve the use of residual skills. The detection of malingering can be very difficult but its essence lies in uncovering the deceit of the patient and leaving him with a certain knowledge that his false symptoms have been recognized. If this goal is achieved, it is common for patients either to discontinue attendance at the clinic, to drop claims for compensation or settle for a low figure and, after a suitable interval, recover and return to work.

Every patient in pain undergoes a change in emotion and many patients with emotional disorders experience pain. Therefore it is important that all those dealing with individuals in pain make themselves competent in the examination of both the patient's physical and psychosocial state.

Recommended reading

1. Bond, M. (1984). *Pain*, 2nd Edn. (Edinburgh: Churchill Livingstone)
2. Merskey, H (1983). Psychological treatment of pain. In Swerdlow, M. (ed.) *Relief of Intractable Pain*, 3rd Edn. (Amsterdam: Elsevier Biomedical Press)

PART TWO
The Pain Patient

5

General Considerations

William Noordenbos

Introduction

When a patient complains of pain the physician must use his clinical experience and knowledge of neurophysiology to try to interpret the meaning of this symptom. Clinical manifestations of pain do not always fit into an appropriate or standard pattern. Some aspects may be puzzling but this does not mean that the patient's complaints are groundless. Pain is a symptom and not a disease and every effort must be made to identify the cause by a full history, clinical examination and any necessary investigations.

Categories of pain complaints

There are four main categories into which pain complaints can be divided. The pain may be due to, or associated with:

I   *External events* such as trauma. Here identification of the main cause is usually not difficult but investigation may show that the patient is responding disproportionately to the injury.

II   *Internal events* are the largest group of causes of pain. Pain may arise from (a) ectodermal tissue (such as the skin), (b) mesodermal tissue (musculoskeletal system), (c) endodermal tissue (e.g. the viscera). Noxious stimuli emanating from the underlying pathology activate receptors in the affected tissues to produce a pattern of afferent impulses which the patient interprets as pain. In many cases this is a direct response but sometimes the pain is referred to a site far removed from the causative lesion and is poorly defined. This may obscure recognition of the causative disorder.

III *Lesions of the afferent nervous system* which involve peripheral nerves, the spinal cord, brain stem, thalamus or higher centres. They are often the consequence of trauma, vascular incidents or polyneuropathies. The majority are partial lesions and cause alterations in the skin sensitivity. The patient is only aware of the results of the lesion which he localizes to the relevant dermatomes. The pain may occur spontaneously or with the lightest stimulation which is not normally noxious, for example, the touch of a feather. Symptoms, including pain, may last indefinitely. The nervous system is not intact and modulating factors have become disrupted (see Chapter 2). Pain disorders in this group are often very puzzling and difficult to treat.

IV *Psychological, social or environmental factors.* Patients should only be placed in this group if they do not have symptoms and signs appropriate to groups I, II or III or if the physical findings are of such a minor or trivial nature as to be the primary cause of the complaints, i.e. there is a gross discrepancy between the observable signs and the subjective complaint. In addition, the doctor should be able to demonstrate psychological factors contributing to the level of distress.

It is important that differentiation between these groups is made as early as possible. If factors of more than one group are involved you must decide where emphasis should be put and in which direction further investigation should be undertaken if more specialized tests are possible.

There are many kinds of pain and it can be difficult to get an accurate, detailed description of its nature. There can also be difficulties in communication between the patient and his physician. The official language of the country, like Urdu or Hindi, may differ from the local language, causing further difficulties in expression for the patient. The physician has to be aware of taboos which prevent the patient from expressing his feelings fully. Therefore, knowledge of the cultural pattern of any particular community is essential.

The physician should be aware that examination of patients with chronic pain is time consuming and that appropriate adjustments must be made to allow for this fact in the organization of the clinic or practice. If this is not done the danger arises of yielding to the temptation to take the easy way out and apply symptomatic treatment, that is to make the pain the target instead of considering the primary disease which gives rise to it. This can have disastrous results.

6

History, Clinical Examination and Assessment

Alistair Young

In many patients a detailed history and clinical examination are sufficient to establish the diagnosis. Investigations and special tests are only necessary if they add to the understanding of the problem. Apart from wasting money, over-investigation can also be potentially dangerous. It may lead some patients to attach undue importance to an otherwise insignificant complaint.

A systematic and logical approach should be adopted. This is particularly necessary when there are a number of different and occasionally conflicting symptoms. Some patients have been seen and investigated by other specialists or received treatment which has been unsuccessful. Information from all sources should be considered, because it may save time by eliminating unnecessary enquiries or may help in clarifying the clinical picture. Particular care should be taken to ensure that the condition is not labelled on a false premise. For example not every patient with pain in the distribution of the trigeminal nerve has trigeminal neuralgia. Equally pain in the back of the head is not necessarily occipital neuralgia. Unless all the necessary information is available it is not uncommon for an inaccurate diagnosis to be made with the result that inappropriate treatment is given to the patient.

HISTORY

Patients must be free to express themselves in any way they choose, but it is necessary to have simple guidelines to channel the information into a purposeful and systematic enquiry.

List of questions about the pain

1. Where is the pain?
2. How long has it been present?
3. How did it start?
4. When did it start?
5. Nature of the pain.
6. Duration of pain.
7. Frequency of attacks.
8. What started the pain?
9. Aggravating factors.
10. Alleviating factors.
11. Associated symptoms.
12. Patient's own opinion of the cause of pain.
13. Other factors – age, sex, etc.

1.   *Where is the pain?*

The site of the pain and any radiation must be noted. The patient who complains of pain all over the body, or in one small area, is unlikely to have physical disease. While the site of the pain may occasionally correlate with its source, as for example in the case of headache due to migraine, it is often unrelated. For example, lumbar pain may be referred from a pancreatic neoplasm and abdominal pain may be referred from spinal nerve roots. Atypical radiation of pain should alert the clinician to the possibility of a non-organic cause. Back pain without radiation into the distribution of a branch of the sciatic nerve is unlikely to be due to protrusion of an intervertebral lumbar disc; equally in the case of trigeminal neuralgia, the pain should be confined to the anatomical distribution of that nerve. In contrast, atypical facial pain may be felt in the neck as much as in the face. Pain due to post-herpetic neuralgia is usually limited to the dermatomes involved by the herpes virus. It is important to decide which system is involved; for example, neurological, musculo-skeletal or vascular disease. However emotional and psychological aspects must not be excluded. They are discussed more fully in Chapter 4.

2. *How long has the pain been present?*

The course and time pattern of any pain often has relevance to the underlying cause. For example pain of long duration without physical signs of organic disease is unlikely to be malignant in origin. On the other hand negative findings should not lead to the pain being dismissed as imaginary or psychosomatic. For example in cluster headache (migrainous neuralgia) the significance of the pain is often unrecognized by both patient and doctor in the absence of objective evidence of disease.

3. *How did the pain start?*

The mode of onset is often characteristic. For example the sudden onset of pain in the distribution of the sciatic nerve, with temporary or marked muscular weakness, is often indicative of a disc lesion. A more gradual onset of pain may not be so significant.

4. *When did the pain start?*

The onset of a number of physical disorders is closely linked to the patient's age. For example, migraine usually starts before age 35; trigeminal neuralgia after the age of 40 and is rare before the age of 30; cervical disc disease tends to occur in middle age, ankylosing spondylitis usually starts in the 30s or 40s and post-herpetic neuralgia is confined to older patients.

5. *What is the pain like?*

The nature of pain is an important clue to its origins. In post-herpetic neuralgia there are several elements which may be present in varying proportions; a superficial burning pain, attacks of sharp, stabbing, shooting or pricking pain, and a constant dull background aching pain. The painful area is often hyperaesthetic. Nerve compression usually results in a constant dull ache with occasional bursts of a 'shooting' pain. Numbness and muscle weakness may also be present. On the other hand severe nerve damage presents with burning pain and hyperpathia. Characteristics of vascular pain are described in Chapter 9; those of rheumatic and arthritic conditions in Chapter 8 and neurological pain in Chapter 7.

Patients vary in their descriptions of pain and their responses to it. For example headache described as a constant tight band suggests muscle tension as the underlying cause but lurid and bizarre presentations without supporting evidence of organic disease are usually due to an emotional complaint. Nevertheless there are exceptions, as for example, thalamic pain which is frequently described as burning in a limb which feels cold. Another unusual presentation is pain felt like knives inserted into the leg and this may be an indication of Tabes Dorsalis. Pain of rheumatoid arthritis is often worse in the morning, when it is accompanied by prolonged muscle stiffness. Bone pathology is suggested by pain which is deeply situated, whereas a continuous throbbing often means inflammation.

6. *How long does the pain last?*

Some pain is constant and unremitting and the patient will not admit to a moment free of pain, although willing to say that the intensity of the pain varies. Such pain occurs with post-herpetic neuralgia, but it may also occur when the pain is of psychological origin.

Brief paroxysms of intense pain are characteristic of trigeminal neuralgia, unlike the constant pain of atypical facial pain.

Migraine is an episodic condition but is frequently over-diagnosed because of the failure to recognize that the attacks of pain should not last more than 48 hours. Constant headaches cannot be attributed to migraine.

7. *How often does the pain occur?*

Migrainous headaches rarely last more than 48 hours and seldom occur more than three times a week. In contrast, cluster headaches occur daily for days to several weeks at a time and then there may be remissions lasting for months or even years.

In gastric ulcer, the pain occurs specifically after each meal, whereas in chronic duodenal ulcer pain occurs on fasting and is relieved by food.

The pain associated with rheumatoid arthritis classically occurs every morning and is associated with stiffness, being made worse by rest (see Chapter 8). The pain of gout occurs in paroxysmal attacks which last from a few days to a few weeks.

8. *What started the pain?*

Often there is an easily defined event, such as trauma, surgical treatment, or infection, causing pain. Post-herpetic neuralgia and post-thoracotomy pain are obvious examples. However, the patient may relate pain to an event in life which is not necessarily its real cause. For example, the onset of abdominal pain caused by diverticulitis, may be attributed by the patient to some coincidental dietary indiscretion. It is important to note that patients often attribute pain due to psychological factors to physical causes.

In patients with atypical facial pain the symptoms are often wrongly attributed to dental disease. Removal of teeth may aggravate rather than relieve the pain.

9. *What aggravates the pain?*

It is important to go into considerable detail when trying to determine what may aggravate the pain because the patient's response to this question may not only aid the diagnosis, but also indicate something of the patient's personality and psychological reaction to the pain.

There are several chronic pain conditions in which the patient can consistently identify factors which aggravate the pain. The classical example is trigeminal neuralgia in which touching the face, talking, chewing or even a cold wind, may trigger the pain. In this condition the patient can also frequently identify one particular area of the face which is sensitive to these stimuli. In thoracic outlet syndrome, in which there is often a cervical rib pressing on the brachial plexus, the pain is usually brought on by use of the hand and arm on that side. Many patients with tension headache claim that the pain is aggravated by bright light and noise. Some patients recognize that stress aggravates this type of headache. The patient with a prolapsed lumbar disc usually reports that lifting, bending and coughing aggravate the pain. In lumbosciatic syndrome due to prolapse of an intervertebral disc, the pain is aggravated by a flexion of the spine, whereas in the facet joint syndrome extension of the spine causes pain. An abdominal nerve entrapment gives rise to pain when the abdominal wall (and therefore the rectus sheath) is tensed, as on coughing, twisting or straining. In ankylosing spondylitis aching and stiffness when lying down force the patient to get up and move around. By contrast, in patients with intermittent claudication due to vascular disturbances in the limbs, the pain may become intolerable after walking only a short distance but ease off after resting for a minute or two.

Finally, it should be remembered that raised emotional tension aggravates all forms of pain and that pain levels are increased when patients are depressed.

10. What relieves the pain?

In considering this question, it should be remembered that the intensity of pain does not necessarily bear any relationship to the nature or severity of the underlying disease. Paradoxically the pain of raised intracranial pressure associated with a cerebral tumour may respond quite readily to analgesics, at least initially, whereas the pain of muscle tension headache may be described as intense and unresponsive. Patients should be questioned about medication and other treatments which they have received and the extent to which these provided relief. This may have been achieved simply by change of posture as occurs with disc protrusion or the local application of heat which can be seen in some patients with disease of the gall bladder.

11. What accompanies the pain?

The presence of other symptoms must be noted and the importance of treating the patient as a whole cannot be too strongly emphasized. Apart from symptoms which obviously accompany pain, the patient's general health must be taken into account. For example, patients with chronic pain may report marked weight loss, but this does not necessarily indicate malignant disease; it may reflect the anxiety that the patient is experiencing because of the pain, particularly if his doctor is unable to make a diagnosis.

It is helpful to enquire specifically about a patient's sleep pattern, because early morning wakening is often the first clue to depression which the patient may, in fact, deny. Patients with chronic pain are often on the defensive and may not respond readily to direct questions about their mental state, whereas they are quite willing to talk about a sleep problem. Ischaemic rest pain occurs in the foot and, at first, may be troublesome only at night. In this case the patient wakens during the hours of sleep to obtain relief by getting up and walking about.

12. *What does the patient believe to be the cause of the pain?*

Patients with pain, particularly if it has been longstanding and undiagnosed, often have a fear of cancer or other serious diseases. Quite often they are reluctant to discuss this fear and specific enquiries may reveal their worries. Convincing the patient that he does not have a serious disease often provides great relief. For example some patients are convinced that their pain is related to a traumatic experience and resent that their view has not been accepted.

13. *Other factors*

The sex of the patient can sometimes be helpful in analyzing the problem and reaching a diagnosis because some chronic pain conditions are sex-related. For example, Raynaud's Disease, ankylosing spondylitis and thromboangiitis obliterans are much commoner in men than in women. In contrast, rheumatoid arthritis, trigeminal neuralgia, temporomandibular pain and migraine are all more commonly seen in women, as is psychogenic pain. Detailed history may reveal many symptoms that are unexplained despite intensive investigation. The thick hospital folder may be a help on occasions but at other times it may be a danger in that the patient's persistent complaint may be too readily dismissed as being due to continuation of a past physical condition or to psychological factors. It cannot be too strongly emphasized that patients with previous psychological disorders may sooner or later develop a physical disease and this may not be revealed unless the examination is completely unbiassed.

THE PHYSICAL EXAMINATION

In many cases the history is sufficient to enable a diagnosis to be made, but nevertheless a thorough physical examination must also be performed. The history may direct attention to the system which is most involved and this should be examined in great detail. However in many patients there is also an important emotional or psychological background which must be investigated. Psychosomatic factors are suggested by fluctuating muscle weakness, sensory loss not corresponding to the anatomical distribution and discrepancies in the patient's performance of everyday activities like dressing and eating. They are particularly important when financial compensation is uppermost in the patient's mind. The history and clinical examination are at least as important as the X ray findings. Degenerative changes of the lumbar spine are not uncommon in the elderly and may not necessarily be relevant. Equally a normal X ray picture does not exclude a physical cause for the pain. If possible these examinations should be repeated at intervals, because they not only reassure a patient that he is being carefully looked after, but occasionally they may reveal previously unsuspected disease.

INVESTIGATIONS

The patient's history and examination usually provide sufficient information to make a provisional diagnosis. Confirmation may be gained from relevant simple investigations, such as urinalysis, a blood count, ESR and plain X rays. These tests may be quite sufficient to reassure both the patient and the clinician. Only occasionally will extensive specialized investigation be needed.

PART THREE
Conditions Causing Chronic Pain

7

Neurological Disease

John Loeser

Introduction

We do not yet fully understand why pathology in the nervous system causes chronic pain or why lesions which produce pain in a few patients (such as amputation or herpes zoster) do not cause chronic pain in the majority.

Mechanical pressure on nerve roots or peripheral nerves is very likely to cause pain, as is an inflammatory process. The pain is usually continuous and is exacerbated by movements of the body which cause impingement on the involved nerve or root. Studies of segments of nerve have shown that regenerating or dying axons as well as neuromata are electrically active and are sensitive to mechanical and chemical stimuli at levels far below those required to activate normal axons. Lesions which cause major somatic sensory loss, whether in the peripheral or central nervous system, lead to chronic pain in about ten per cent of patients. These 'central pain states' or 'deafferentation pains' are usually continuous and unrelated to external events. They are often associated with clinical evidence of altered sensory fields. As stimulation of a remote region of the body will result in a sensation in the deafferented area, it seems that there has been reorganisation of central synapses in response to denervation. In some chronic pain states, there is little evidence that the primary pathology involves nerves as, for example, in migraine, cluster headaches, some forms of low back pain and some of the pain syndromes ascribed to visceral dysfunction. Indeed, the roles of affective and environmental factors in chronic pain must always be considered.

CAUSES OF NEUROLOGICAL PAIN

Tables 1, 2 and 3 detail the causes of neurological pain.

Table 1   Facial pain

Common causes:	Trigeminal neuralgia
	Atypical facial pain
	Vascular neuralgias
Others:	Myofascial
	Inflammation – paranasal sinuses
	Temporal arteritis
	Temporo-mandibular joint dysfunction
	Peripheral neuropathies – e.g. diabetes mellitus

Table 2   Headache

Muscle tension
Migraine
Referred e.g. cervical arthritis
Temporal arteritis
Hypertension
Sinusitis
Miscellaneous – No identifiable cause

Table 3   Spinal cord and nerve root pain

Spinal cord lesions
Multiple sclerosis
Radicular pain
   Nerve root compression – e.g. I.V. disc
   Inflammatory – e.g. Post-herpetic neuralgia
   Neoplastic
Arachnoiditis – e.g. following trauma, surgery, myelography
Spinal stenosis
Post-paraplegic pain
Peripheral nerve lesions–Nerve roots or plexus
Polyneuropathies
Autonomic nervous system – e.g. Reflex sympathetic dystrophy

FACIAL PAIN

There are three common types of facial pain that are of neurological origin:

1. Trigeminal neuralgia
2. Atypical facial pain
3. Vascular facial neuralgia.

These must be differentiated from the other causes of facial pain which are described on page 65 et seq.

Trigeminal neuralgia (tic douloureux)

This is a unique pain syndrome with the characteristic features of severe electric shock-like stabbing pains. The attacks are of sudden onset and equally abrupt termination and the patient is pain free in between. The pain is always unilateral, but a few patients have a history of previous attacks on the opposite side. The pain is triggered by non-noxious stimulation from the ipsilateral peri-oral region or from other more distal sites. The pain is usually restricted to the distribution of the trigeminal nerve but in a small percentage of patients the pain involves the glossopharyngeal or nervus intermedius territories. Trigeminal neuralgia is most common in the elderly, but it can occur at any age. It is slightly more frequent in women than men.

Episodes of pain may occur at varying intervals and in some patients years elapse between attacks. When the pain has been active for a year without remission there is little chance of spontaneous improvement. The vast majority of patients have an aberrant blood vessel (usually the superior cerebellar artery) impinging on the trigeminal root just as it leaves the pons. When the pain is in the glossopharyngeal distribution the offending artery is found at the root entry zone of that nerve.

The management of trigeminal neuralgia is primarily pharmacological. Phenytoin and carbamazepine when properly used are effective in about two-thirds of the patients (see also Chapter 12). When drug therapy fails to control the pain or when the patient develops intolerable side effects a surgical procedure should be considered. Percutaneous trigeminal gangliolysis either with a radiofrequency probe or glycerol injection is the safest and most effective method of partially destroying the nerve and controlling the pain. Gangliolysis has supplanted alcohol injection and peripheral neurectomy as the elective procedure. It has an 80% one year and 60% five year success rate. The complication rate is less than one half per cent. Suboccipital craniectomy with decompression of the trigeminal nerve appears to have an 80% five year success rate; it does not lead to any facial numbness; the complication rate is about 5%. (For details of technique see Recommended Reading).

Atypical facial pain

Atypical facial pain usually occurs in young adults, much more commonly in women than men. It is characterised by continuous, burning, aching pain which may be unilateral or bilateral and may overflow the territory of the trigeminal nerve into the cervical dermatomes. There is often a complaint of numbness or distortion of sensation in the painful area and the pain is exacerbated by stimulation of this area. Unlike patients with trigeminal neuralgia those with atypical facial pain frequently have a pre-existing history of psychological and behavioural dysfunction. They are difficult patients to manage and may commit suicide. Intensity of pain fluctuates with stimulation or stress, and it does not start and stop suddenly like trigeminal neuralgia.

Patients who have bilateral atypical facial pain are very unlikely to have a pathological disorder and do not respond to any form of medical or surgical therapy. Indeed, they are uniformly made worse by any procedure which denervates the painful area, in spite of the fact that a local anaesthetic will temporarily stop the pain. Intra-oral burning pain is a similar syndrome which plagues dentists; these patients are almost always female.

Unilateral atypical facial pain

Unilateral atypical facial pain must be thoroughly evaluated because a small percentage of patients have a structural lesion affecting the trigeminal nerve or deep structures at the base of the skull. The presence of progressive sensory loss should increase suspicion that such a lesion is present. Unilateral atypical facial pain may follow injury to a branch of the trigeminal nerve such as after dental surgery. In a few patients there is a tumour invading the base of the skull or in the retropharyngeal space. This type of pain is also seen after infarction in the medulla involving the trigeminal tract and nucleus (usually in the distribution of the posterior inferior cerebellar artery).

Progressive sensory loss over a period of time in a consistent dermatomal pattern is almost certainly due to a neoplasm impinging on the trigeminal nerve.

There are many variants of atypical facial pain: the outcome from either medical or surgical therapy is better the more the disease resembles classical trigeminal neuralgia. The management of atypical facial pain is unsatisfactory but a combination of a tricyclic anti-depressant with a phenothiazine may provide relief in some cases. On rare occasions an anticonvulsant drug proves helpful. Surgery is rarely effective unless structural pathology is present. Psychiatric treatment also does not seem to alleviate this type of pain. Fortunately, atypical facial pain gradually lessens in severity over a few years, or alternatively, the patient recognizes that physicians have little to offer and the complaints gradually dwindle. It should be obvious that narcotics and sedative-hypnotic medications have no place in the management of this chronic pain state.

Vascular facial pain

Vascular facial pains and anterior head pains are a distinct group of chronic pains which come in many varieties. They are usually characterised by burning, dysaesthetic sensations associated with lacrimation, rhinitis, flushing and sweating of the face. The pain often builds to a crescendo over ten to thirty minutes and lasts for a few hours. It is virtually always unilateral and involves the maxillary and retro-orbital regions more than the mandibular and ophthalmic. The pains characteristically come in clusters (hence the common name of 'cluster headache') which are not triggered and are not associated with sensory loss. The painful area may be tender to palpation. It is much more common in males than females and is most prevalent in young adults. There is rarely a positive family history; no associated neurological diseases have been recognized. The management of cluster headaches is pharmacological (see Chapter 12).

Other facial pains

The differential diagnosis of facial pains must include the consideration of some syndromes which are not primarily of neurological origin. These include temporo-mandibular joint dysfunction, which usually produces lateral face pain which may radiate to the jaw or temple; myofascial syndrome involving the muscles of mastication, which usually produces local pain and tenderness to palpation; temporal arteritis, which is responsible for pain over the superficial temporal artery and is associated with an elevated erythrocyte sedimentation rate and tumour or infection in the paranasal sinuses or jaws which produces local pain and X-ray changes.

HEADACHES

Headaches are common but fortunately most are short-lived and spontaneously improve. Few patients develop a chronic headache which is severe enough to disrupt daily life. The common forms of headache are those due to muscle tension in the posterior cervical muscles, migraine, referred pain from cervical arthritis, temporal arteritis, hypertension and sinusitis.

Migraine

Migraine can be conveniently divided into classic, common and complicated varieties.

Classic migraine

Classic migraine is produced by hemiparesis, hemisensory deficit, vertigo or other neurological abnormalities. The aura usually lasts ten to twenty minutes and gradually abates as the headache begins. Most patients report a focal origin of their headache on one side of the scalp or frontal area; the pain then generalizes and becomes throbbing. Each headache usually lasts for many hours and the patient is obviously ill. Classic migraine usually has its onset in adolescence; the frequency of attacks varies from several a week to a few in a lifetime. A wide variety of allergies, stresses and hormonal cycling have been identified as precipitating factors and there is definitely a genetic predisposition to the disease.

Common migraine

This is similar in many ways to classic migraine but is not characterized by a pre-headache aura. However vague warning signs may be noted by the patient. The headache itself is usually most intense behind the eye and is often said to be throbbing. Patients often describe lacrimation and nasal stuffiness; this type of headache is similar to cluster headaches in this respect. Common migraine headache often begins while the patient is asleep or early in the morning and occurs after, rather than during, stressful events.

Complicated migraine

This rare form of migraine headache is characterized by the development of a major neurological deficit which begins at the same time as the headache and usually outlasts it, often by hours or days. The two commonest varieties are hemiplegic and ophthalmoplegic migraine; some families will manifest both forms. A patient with complicated migraine requires full neurological assessment to rule out a structural lesion.

The management of migraine is by drug treatment which is usually but not always successful (see Chapter 13).

Muscle tension headache

This common type of headache often starts in adolescence and varies in frequency and intensity. Most patients report that they awaken without headache and that their pain begins in the afternoon or early evening. The pain may be unilateral or bilateral and radiates from the suboccipital region over or around the head of the frontal area. There are no associated neurological signs or symptoms. Emotional stress is clearly a precipitating factor. Prior neck injury, especially a minor injury, is sometimes identified by the patient as a causative factor. The pain is described as aching, cramping, rarely throbbing; the skin of the neck and scalp may be dysaesthetic. There is often tenderness of the posterior cervical musculature in general and the region of the greater occipital nerves as they pierce the trapezius muscle. Other causes of similar pain are cervical arthritis and myofascial syndromes involving the muscles of mastication, both of which can cause referred pain. The patient should be assured that there is no significant intracranial pathology. Management consists of the use of local physical measures, such as heat, cold, vibration and massage which are often helpful. Correction of posture when sitting to avoid fixed and awkward positions of the neck also helps. Drugs should be limited to the use of an agent like aspirin. Narcotics and sedative-hypnotic drugs must be avoided. Relief of emotional stress will also help.

Increased intracranial pressure headache

Increased intracranial pressure due to any cause can produce chronic headache. The usual history is of relentless, increasingly severe, diffuse throbbing or aching pain. It is usually worse in the morning or when lying down and is often aggravated by bending or straining. The appearance of a progressive neurological abnormality in a patient with headache indicates the need for investigation.

Headaches can also be part of the poorly understood and uncommon syndrome labelled 'benign intracranial hypertension'. This usually occurs in young adult women who are overweight, but can occur in either sex at any age. It may, in some cases, be precipitated by the use of topical steroids. The patient complains of diffuse headache, worse in the morning or when lying down. Papilloedema and visual changes are common. High doses of steroids (dexamethasone 4 mg) every 6 hours usually provide relief of the headache and visual changes; the syndrome seems to abate spontaneously over months and long term therapy is usually required.

Temporal arteritis headache

Temporal arteritis often produces unilateral temporal headache (see Chapter 9 and Recommended Reading).

Other causes of headache

A wide variety of drugs, chemicals and toxins can lead to both acute and chronic headache. Almost one-half of the patients with systemic hypertension have some degree of headache; but whether or not this is due to the elevation of blood pressure is uncertain. Severe hypertension (diastolic pressure > 120 mm Hg) is uniformly associated with chronic headache which may fluctuate as the blood pressure changes due to position or exertion. Effective control of the hypertension is the primary method of managing this type of pain.

SPINAL CORD AND NERVE ROOT PAIN SYNDROMES

Many diseases which affect the spinal cord and nerve roots can lead to chronic pain. The history and localization of the lesion will suggest the likely cause. Most diseases which are restricted to the spinal cord itself (myelopathies) do not lead to pain but are much more likely to cause loss of normal sensations. Radiculopathies, in contrast, are much more likely to cause pain and sensory or motor changes which are relatively focal.

Spinal cord lesions causing pain

Multiple sclerosis can cause signs and symptoms due to spinal cord involvement. Occasionally pain is the presenting symptom, characterized by exacerbations and remissions of neurological signs throughout the central nervous system. Burning, dysaesthetic pains are the most common, but electric-shock like pains, paraesthesiae and hyperpathia also occur. The distribution of the pains may be dermatomal or regional depending on the site of the demyelinating lesion.

Nerve root lesions causing pain

The posterior nerve root and spinal ganglion are extremely sensitive to mechanical deformation; these are the most common sites of painful processes involving the spinal column or its contents. The spasms arising from or impinging on the posterior roots at any level will often cause a radicular pain which radiates from the midline into the involved dermatome.

Inflammatory diseases or inflammatory responses to bacterial or viral infection are other causes of radicular pain. The lightning pains of tabes dorsalis (tertiary syphilis) are an example, as is post-herpetic neuralgia. Arachnoiditis following infection, trauma, surgery or myelography with oil-based media probably causes pain by its involvement of the dorsal roots. Post-herpetic neuralgia can affect any part of the body but is commonest in the face and thoracic regions. The acute phase of this disease is always painful: Inflammatory changes occur in the dorsal roots and extend into the spinal cord. Older patients are much more likely to develop post-herpetic neuralgia. Pharmacological therapy in the chronic phase is not very effective but some patients will benefit from the combination of a tricyclic antidepressant and a phenothiazine. Anticonvulsant medications may help if the pain is chiefly shooting or stabbing in nature. The shooting pains of tabes dorsalis usually respond to treatment with carbamazepine.

Nerve root compression

Mechanical pressure on the nerve root by a ruptured or bulging disc or stenosis of the neural canal or the nerve root foramen is a cause of back and radicular pain in a small proportion of patients with back or neck pain. Nerve root compression can also be due to impingement in the neural foramen by osteophytes or hypertrophied facet joints. Nerve root compression is fully discussed in Chapter 8.

Spinal stenosis

This condition of narrowing of the spinal canal can cause pain and neurological dysfunction in the lower limbs which is made worse by walking (neurogenic claudication). This can be a congenital lesion or may be due to degenerative changes in the spine. The only treatment for spinal stenosis which is causing serious disability is surgical decompression.

Post-paraplegic pain

About five per cent of the patients who sustain a major spinal cord injury develop a chronic pain syndrome which may be due to one of three causes: unstable fracture site, nerve root compression by bone or disc fragment and injury to the spinal cord. The presence of radicular pain which is exacerbated by movement suggests nerve root compression. Confirmation of the lesion is by X-rays in flexion and extension which show movement at the level of injury. The patient who reports a burning, aching pain below the level of his sensory deficits which is constant and not related to activity probably has *deafferentation pain* which is not likely to respond to pharmacological treatment or surgery.

PERIPHERAL NERVE PAIN SYNDROMES

Pain can be due to mechanical pressure, inflammation or demyeliniz-ation in nerve plexuses or peripheral nerves. Plexus lesions and mono-neuropathies are local disorders in contrast to polyneuropathies which are diffuse conditions usually secondary to metabolic or toxic factors.

Pain due to a lesion of plexus or peripheral nerve may be sharp and stabbing, a continuous burning and aching or a combination of both. There does not appear to be any relationship between the causative agent and the nature of the pain, although pains associated with significant sensory loss are more likely to be of the burning, dysaesthetic variety. The distribution of pain is not usually restricted to the site of the lesion but tends to extend into the superficial or deep sensory field of the involved nerve. The findings on physical examination can be corroborated by X-rays to locate bony lesions compressing peripheral nerves or a plexus.

In focal disorders of the peripheral nervous system, it is important to determine if movement aggravates or reproduces the patient's pain. If a nerve is compressed by a mass or entrapped by muscle or a fascial band, direct pressure over the site will usually increase the pain. If there has been degeneration and then regeneration of axons, tapping the nerve at any point distal to the compressed area will cause the patient to complain of paraesthesiae (Tinel's Sign). Mechanical manoeuvres such as wrist flexion increase the signs of median nerve entrapment in the carpal tunnel (Phelan's Sign). Straight-leg raising to stretch the sciatic nerve and its roots can also help in the identification of nerve compression at specific regions.

Brachial plexus pain syndromes

Brachial plexus lesions often cause pain in the neck, shoulder and arm on the same side. The pain may be increased by neck or limb movements or by deep breathing. Light pressure over the region of the plexus in the root of the neck may reproduce the patient's pain. The condition is usually due to local trauma – for example, stab wounds or hyper-extension stretching injuries as occur in motor cycle accidents. There is often severe pain at the time of injury, but even more debilitating, chronic, burning, dysaesthetic pain may follow. The management of brachial plexus pain is difficult; a few patients may respond to anticonvulsant drugs or the combination of a tricyclic antidepressant and a phenothiazine. Some special neurosurgical techniques may bring pain relief but amputation must not be performed because it will not relieve pain and may indeed make it worse.

Thoracic outlet syndrome

This usually involves the lower trunk (C8-T1 roots) of the plexus and is due to compression of the nerves by muscle or bone. Pain may be referred in the entire shoulder and arm or may be specific to the involved segments. Sensory and motor changes may occur and vascular compression (subclavian or axillary artery) can also be significant. There can be no question that this syndrome exists in some patients, particularly those with a cervical rib, scalene spasm or abnormal fascial bands, but this diagnosis is far too frequently made.

Lumbosacral plexus lesions

Lesions of the lumbosacral plexus are much less common than those of the brachial plexus. As in the upper extremity, plexus lesions are usually unilateral; bilateral lesions suggest spinal cord or cauda equina involvement. Damage to the lumbosacral plexus will only occur if there is major pelvic trama or a penetrating injury. Pregnancy and childbirth are associated with a variety of injuries to the plexus which can cause chronic pain. For example, the foetal head can compress the plexus; traumatic delivery can produce a severe injury, usually to the sacral components. Haemorrhage and infection in the retroperitoneal space can lead to chronic pain due to inflammatory changes within the plexus.

Peripheral nerve lesions

All the peripheral nerves in the extremities are subject to entrapment syndromes which can cause chronic pain and loss of sensory and motor function. Sometimes the sensory and motor loss is minimal and pain is the major complaint; sympathetic nerve function may also be affected leading to skin temperature and sweating changes. In the arm, the two most common sites are the ulnar nerve at the elbow and the median nerve at the wrist (*carpal tunnel syndrome*). In the leg, entrapment of the sciatic nerve by the pyriformis muscle can occur in the buttock, the peroneal nerve at the fibular head, the interdigital nerves in the foot or the posterior tibial nerve in the tarsal tunnel. The lateral femoral cutaneous nerve can also be compressed (*meralgia paraesthetica*).

Other causes of painful neuropathy include compression by neoplasms, local infection and diabetic vasculopathy leading to nerve infarction.

After a peripheral nerve has been cut there may be a localized pain due to the formation of a neuroma. A neuroma is often extremely sensitive to local pressure and temperature changes. Treatment with analgesic drugs is only of short-term benefit. However, surgical repair of a damaged nerve may abolish neuroma pain. Resection of the neuroma is unlikely to help; but a more valuable procedure is transposition of the neuroma to a less sensitive area. It is important to point out that pain syndromes related to nerve injuries and deafferentation are at least partly due to changes in the central nervous system. Some pain states depend on a combination of peripheral and central mechanisms and are then not responsive to peripheral (i.e. interruption of transmission) techniques alone.

Phantom limb pain persists in 5–10% of people who lose the whole or part of a limb. It almost never occurs in children and is much more common in the elderly. This type of pain must be distinguished from stump pain. The patient describes a painfully distorted and often foreshortened limb; occasionally there are sharp intermittent pains as well as a constant cramping and aching sensation. No form of therapy is very successful but electrical stimulation of the peripheral nerve or spinal cord is sometimes useful. Anticonvulsant medication may reduce shooting pain and the combination of a tricyclic antidepressant and a phenothiazine may relieve the cramping pain. Simple analgesics are unhelpful.

Causalgia

Causalgia is a constant burning pain associated with signs of autonomic dysfunction: loss of sweating, vasodilation or vasoconstriction and trophic changes in skin, muscle and joints. It is always associated with a partial or occasionally complete injury to a mixed peripheral nerve, usually the median or sciatic. The patient is in agony and refuses to move or touch the painful part. If untreated, causalgia results in total loss of function in the damaged extremity. Prompt performance of sympathetic nerve block or intravenous regional perfusion (see Chapter 13), accompanied by intensive physical therapy will usually reverse the symptoms.

Reflex sympathetic dystrophy

Reflex sympathetic dystrophy is in many ways similar to causalgia but does not follow a peripheral nerve injury. Instead, trauma to bone or joint seems to be the precipitating factor. Excruciating pain develops over days following the injury; the patient refuses to use the involved limb and secondary changes of disuse atrophy are superimposed upon the autonomic dysfunction. Again, sympathetic blocks and physical therapy if initiated early are very likely to bring relief.

Polyneuropathies

Peripheral polyneuropathies are characterized by symmetrical bilateral alterations in sensation and motor function which are more marked distally. The sensory loss does not follow the territory of any peripheral nerve or dermatome. Lower extremities are usually more involved than the upper. Although pain may be a major complaint, it is not usually the first symptom noted by the patient. Varying degrees of sensory loss, motor loss and pain may be present and do not seem to correlate well with either the aetiological agent or the neuropathological changes in the nerve. Some patients complain of a diffuse cramping pain which is worse when they are inactive; this may lead to the *'restless legs syndrome'*. A larger percentage of patients complain of hyperpathia in the regions of hypaesthesia. Dysaesthesia and paraesthesia are common complaints.

Polyneuropathies are almost always due to a toxic or metabolic insult. Diabetes mellitus is a common underlying disease; other diagnostic possibilities include alcoholic neuropathy, organophosphorus neuropathy and a variety of metabolic disorders, porphyria, etc. Most polyneuropathies are not characterized by severe pain, but some patients are greatly disabled. Polyneuropathies rarely produce areas of normal and abnormal sensation; such a finding should raise the question of a functional disorder. The management of the pain of a polyneuropathy is initially based upon treatment of the underlying metabolic or toxic abnormality; anticonvulsant and/or antidepressant medications are sometimes helpful.

Recommended reading

Matthews, W.B. and Miller, H. (1976). *Diseases of the Nervous System*, 2nd Edn. (Oxford: Blackwell)
White, J.C. and Sweet, W.H. (1969). *Pain and Neurosurgeon*. (Springfield, IL: Charles C. Thomas)

8

Musculo-skeletal and Rheumatic Disease

Malcolm Jayson

Introduction

The management of musculo-skeletal or rheumatic disorders depends upon diagnosis of the underlying condition and assessment of the nature, severity and extent of musculo-skeletal damage. General pain relieving measures applied alone will provide little benefit and will allow the underlying disorder to persist untreated. As a rule successful treatment requires a careful management programme. Therapy is directed at the underlying disorder and pure pain relieving procedures are reserved for those patients for whom it is not possible to obtain adequate relief of the causal condition.

This chapter deals with the comon forms of musculo-skeletal disease and in particular chronic inflammatory polyarthritis, back pain and various forms of soft tissue rheumatism. Infections, neoplasms and metabolic disorders of bone are not included except as differential diagnoses. Clearly it is essential to recognise their presence and to provide appropriate treatment.

CHRONIC INFLAMMATORY POLYARTHRITIS

This is a large group of conditions in which chronic inflammation develops in several joints and persists producing pain and disability. Cultures of the synovial fluid and the synovium are sterile. There is proliferation of the lining of the joint which may lead to erosion of the articular surfaces and the development of permanent joint damage.

The most common of these disorders is rheumatoid arthritis. Its management has formed the basis for development of anti-inflammatory drugs and the management of other rheumatic problems. Careful assessment is required to differentiate other diseases, mentioned on page 77.

Rheumatoid arthritis

There is usually a chronic symmetrical peripheral inflammatory polyarthritis which is often associated with joint erosions seen on X-rays, subcutaneous nodules and positive tests for rheumatoid factor.

Clinical features

Rheumatoid arthritis occurs in approximately 1 per cent of males and 2–3 per cent of females. It is found throughout the world although it seems to develop particularly as a disease of civilization and is relatively rare in primitive communities. Its pathogenesis is uncertain. There are clear genetic factors and an important association with the tissue type HLA-DR4. Autoimmune changes are common and may play a pathogenic role and possibly certain infective organisms such as viruses initiate development of this disorder.

The disease may develop insidiously with aches and pains and transient swelling of one or two joints. As it progresses clear features of synovitis develop in multiple joints. The patient develops pain and stiffness and characteristically these symptoms are exacerbated by rest particularly at night with a marked element of morning stiffness. Involved joints become swollen and painful and examination shows the presence of increased temperature, tenderness on palpation, synovial thickening and effusion. With progress of the disease deformities and limitation of movement occur.

Rheumatoid arthritis can affect any synovial joint. Most frequently it involves the metocarpophalangeal and proximal interphalangeal joints of the fingers, the wrists and the metatarsophalangeal joints of the toes. Less frequently it affects the elbows, knees, shoulders, hips and neck.

In certain sites (in particular the hands) the tendon sheaths are lined by synovium. Synovitis may affect these tendon sheaths. This is common and in early rheumatoid arthritis limitation of hand function is more commonly due to tenosynovitis than to joint disease. Careful examination is required as tendon sheath involvement is easily missed.

With progress of the disease there are certain characteristic patterns of deformities and disabilities. In the hands common problems are ulnar deviation at the metacarpophalangeal joints, swan neck and 'button hole' deformities of the fingers. Rupture of the tendons on the dorsal surface of the wrist may cause 'dropped' fingers. In the feet a common problem is dorsal subluxation of the toes with the fatty pad normally under the metatarsal heads slipping forwards leaving the bones unprotected. Patients complain of severe pain under the forefeet and describe the sensation as 'walking on stones'.

Complications

Rhematoid arthritis is a systemic disorder with multiple extra-articular features. Some may be a consequence of treatment. In particular drug therapy may cause blood dyscrasias and gastrointestinal problems.

Seronegative polyarthritis

This is a group of disorders which form part of a complex disease pattern and frequently show many overlapping features. The principal disorders to be considered are:

1. Ankylosing spondylitis
2. Psoriatic arthritis
3. Reiter's syndrome and reactive arthritis
4. The arthritis of ulcerative colitis and Crohn's disease

Features which are common to these disorders are inflammatory peripheral polyarthritis, sacroiliitis and spondylitis, negative tests for rheumatoid factor and an association with the tissue type HLA B27. This tissue type occurs in about 5 to 8 per cent of the normal population but in 95 per cent of patients with ankylosing spondylitis, 90 per cent of those with Reiter's syndrome and in 40 to 60 per cent of the patients in the other three groups. There appear to be important genetic factors predisposing towards the development of these conditions and the exact pattern may be determined by precipitating factors such as bowel or urogenital infections.

Ankylosing spondylitis

This is a common disorder more frequently appearing in men, aged between 15 and 25 years, but which is almost as common in women.

Inflammation usually develops in the sacroiliac joints and spine but also elsewhere, causing pain and stiffness, and may be followed by ossification of the spinal ligaments producing rigidity and deformity.

It usually starts with low back pain and stiffness which are aggravated by rest and relieved by exercise. The patient wakes in the early morning and obtains relief by a few simple exercises. At first the back may appear normal, but as the disease advances stiffness lasts for longer periods and eventually becomes permanent. The patient may develop a characteristic posture with loss of the normal lumbar lordosis and a smooth dorsal kyphosis. The neck is often hyperextended so the patient can look forward. In severe cases, localized pain may develop in the back due to excessive movement at any remaining mobile segment. This may be related to trauma as the fused spine is brittle and fractures can occur readily.

The disease may be complicated by a peripheral inflammatory arthritis usually in the lower limbs. It is less severe than rheumatoid arthritis but involved hips may rapidly lose movements and ankylose. The combination of fused spine and ankylosed hips produces very severe disability.

Ankylosing spondylitis is associated with recurrent iritis and with chronic inflammatory bowel disease such as ulcerative colitis and Crohn's disease.

Reactive arthritis (Reiter's syndrome)

Reiter's syndrome most commonly develops as a venereally acquired disease but it may also follow dysenteric diseases such as Shigella and Salmonella enteritis or infection by other organisms. The syndrome is known as 'reactive arthritis'.

Characteristic features include a non-specific urethritis followed by conjunctivitis and arthritis. The arthritis predominantly involves the lower limbs with inflammatory changes in the joints of the toes, the tarsus, ankles and knees. A rash occurs on the soles of the feet and elsewhere and resembles pustular psoriasis. Patients may develop ulcers in the mouth and other problems.

The initial attack usually remits but relapses may lead to severe joint damage and involve the spine to produce changes of ankylosing spondylitis.

Arthritis of ulcerative colitis (*Crohn's disease*)

Patients with Crohn's disease may develop an inflammatory arthritis, predominantly in the lower limbs but sometimes presenting as sacroiliitis and ankylosing spondylitis. The severity of the peripheral arthritis is related to the degree of activity of the colitis so that control of the inflammatory bowel disease may be required to relieve the arthritis.

Management of chronic inflammatory arthritis

The principles of treatment are similar for the various disorders with specific variations for the individual diseases and their problems. They involve the various modalities listed in Table 1. The vast majority of patients are managed in a conservative fashion with rest, physiotherapy, non-steroidal anti-inflammatory drugs and environmental adjustments; few require more active or invasive forms of treatment.

Table 1   Principles of management of chronic inflammatory arthritis

Rest–	Bed, splints
Physiotherapy–	Pain relief – ultrasonics, short wave etc.
	Rehabilitation – exercises, training
Occupational therapy–	Aids, environmental adjustments, training
Non-steroidal anti-inflammatory drugs	
Anti-rheumatic drugs–	Gold, penicillamine, chloroquine
Corticosteroids	
Immuno-suppressive agents	
Intra-articular injections	
Surgery	

Rest

In acute *rheumatoid arthritis* bed rest may be helpful in promoting remissions of the disease. It is important that inflamed joints are rested in a neutral position as flexion deformities develop all too readily. In particular splints should be provided for hands, fingers and also for the knees. It is far easier to prevent deformities than to correct them once they have occurred. Established disabilities might have been prevented if appropriate splinting and other corrective measures had been applied at the right time.

Physiotherapy

The primary role of physiotherapy is to strengthen muscle power and improve function by maintaining or increasing the range of joint movement and activity. Exercises are a basic requirement and should be isometric when there is inflammation, with active mobilization only when synovitis is quiescent. The physiotherapist will need to help with this regime when the arthritis is active but, as the patient improves, he can perform them on his own and even exercise against resistance. Heat (from a short wave diathermy machine, radiant lamp or a wax bath), massage or ice packs sometimes temporarily relieve pain and may encourage early movement but they make no difference to the long term result.

Spinal mobilization and exercise are most important in ankylosing spondylitis and should be performed daily. At the same time careful attention is directed to posture and the prevention of spinal deformities and rigidity. As the arthritis remits patients should be encouraged to return to normal activity. They may need to learn again how to get out of a chair, walk and climb stairs. It is better to do these activities gradually, rest in the afternoon for example and conserve energies for the rest of the day. The reeducation programe should not be pushed beyond the patient's endurance.

Occupational therapy

There are a number of aids and appliances which take the strain away from damaged or infected joints. Some are concerned with feeding, washing, dressing and other domestic activities. Patients must learn from a skilled therapist how to use these, so that they can rehabilitate themselves for an early return to work and normal living.

Pharmacological therapy

1. *Non-steroid anti-inflammatory drugs (NSAIDs)*

These drugs are described in Chapter 12.

2. *Anti-rheumatoid drugs*

Gold

Gold is undoubtedly a valuable therapeutic agent in rheumatoid arthritis, but because of toxicity about a third of the patients who are treated with it have to be withdrawn and put onto alternative regimes.

d-Penicillamine

d-Penicillamine or dimethylcysteine is the D-isomer derived by hydrolysis of penicillin. Like gold it produces remissions of rheumatoid arthritis usually after a couple of months but it can also produce toxic complications.

Penicillamine is usually given in an initial dose of 125 mg daily and then increased by similar amounts at 3 to 4 week intervals until the patient goes into remission, or until a maximum dose of 750 mg or perhaps 1000 mg per day is reached. If remission is not achieved at the largest dose then the drug should be withdrawn. Penicillamine should be taken at least one and a half hours after meals or other drugs and one and a half hours before the next meal. Toxic reactions are not uncommon.

3. *Anti-malarials*

Chloroquine produces remissions of rheumatoid arthritis after two to three months of treatment. This drug does not seem as effective as gold or penicillamine but the relative ease of its use may make it more appropriate. Chloroquine is used in a dose of 250 mg per day. The principal toxic effects are on the eyes; the drug can be deposited in the retina and may lead to a retinopathy.

4. *Corticosteroids*

Corticosteroids have dramatic anti-inflammatory properties but unfortunately their side effects commonly outweigh the clinical advantages. Their use should be strictly reserved for the most difficult problems. The gluco-corticoids, e.g. prednisolone, are used in the lowest possible dose and every effort should be made to reduce the total amount taken during long term therapy. In uncomplicated rheumatoid arthritis the maximum dose of prednisolone should not be more than 5 to 7.5 mg per day and preferably less. Even on these doses in the long term serious complications may arise. Short sharp courses of corticosteroids should not be used. Too often it proves impossible to withdraw the steroids and patients may be committed to long term treatment when it has not been strictly necessary. In rheumatoid arthritis the indications for steroid therapy are as follows:

1. Persistent active inflammation in multiple joints despite a proper course of more conservative therapy.

2. Systemic complications such as pericarditis or vasculitis.

3. In less severe cases of joint inflammation because of important work or domestic problems.

Steroids are also used for seronegative polyarthritis, connective tissue disorders like systemic lupus erythematosus, dermatomyositis, polymyalgia rheumatica and polyarteritis nodosa. Careful assessment is required in every case.

Side effects with steroid therapy are dyspepsia, peptic ulceration, osteoporosis, vertebral fractures and dermal atrophy. In children growth may be retarded and so steroids should be restricted to minimal dosage on alternate days. When there are complications steroid intake may need to be reduced, preferably gradually or by changing to an alternate day regime. In some cases supplementary therapy with immunosuppressive drugs is helpful. However even when steroids have been stopped the hypopituitary-adrenal axis may be inadequate to cope with additional stress or infection for three years after their withdrawal. Patients should carry a card indicating they have been on steroids, so that appropriate supplements can be given in the event of extra demands due to stress or intercurrent infection (see Recommended Reading).

Intra-articular therapy

Intra-articular injection of slow release preparations containing corticosteroids often induces remission in the synovitis affecting that joint. Hydrocortisone acetate is the least expensive but other preparations such as methyl prednisolone acetate have more prolonged actions.

Local steroid injections are particularly indicated when the general inflammation is coming under control but smouldering activity is still present in one or two joints or tendon sheaths. There may be difficulty in flexing individual fingers or perhaps a trigger finger indicating palmar tenosynovitis. This responds to local injection therapy as does median nerve compression in the carpal tunnel syndrome. The injection must be given into the sheath of the tendon but not into its substance, otherwise it may rupture. Fluorinated compounds like triamcinolone are liable to produce fat atrophy and should not be used for superficial injections.

Scrupulous asepsis must be observed during the performance of these injections because there is a high risk of infection. The procedure should be abandoned if there is any suspicion of the joint or tendon sheath being infected. In some cases this may mean preliminary aspiration and culture of the fluid withdrawn. It is possible to inject more than one site at the same time but systemic absorption of the steroid can produce general problems. Repeated injections may be performed at intervals but multiple injections into a single joint may lead to joint damage.

Surgery

New developments in joint surgery have produced dramatic changes in the prognosis of patients with chronic inflammatory arthritis. It is now possible to restore function and relieve pain for many who would previously have been severely disabled. Decisions are best made by the physician and surgeon together to assess the medical and surgical problems and plan the treatment programme.

In general surgery can be divided into soft tissue procedures, such as synovectomy and tenosynovectomy which are aimed at preventing joint and tendon damage and relieving pressure on damaged nerves, and reconstructive surgery which is directed at restoring function.

A variety of procedures may be performed on the hands. In the wrist carpal tunnel decompression relieves the symptoms and signs of median nerve compression. Tenosynovectomy may be performed for involvement of the flexor or extensor tendons. For wrist problems, resection of the ulnar styloid may relieve pain and improve grip strength and in severe cases arthrodesis of the wrist is helpful. Damaged metacarpophalangeal joints can be replaced with relief of pain but limited improvement in function. For active synovitis involving the elbow, synovectomy (sometimes with resection of the radial head) is useful.

A very common problem in the feet is metatarsophalangeal subluxation with the toes over-riding the metatarsal heads to lie on the dorsum of the foot. The patient develops severe pain beneath the metatarsal heads with formation of callosities and sometimes ulceration. Fusion procedures may be helpful for hind foot and ankle problems. For the knee synovectomy may be performed in early disease; it relieves synovitis but it is uncertain whether it protects the joint against long term damage. Knee replacement has become a very successful operation. The newest designs are aimed at preserving as much of the bone as possible and replacing the articular surfaces.

Hip problems have been revolutionized by low friction total hip replacement.

Crystal induced arthritis

There are a number of forms of acute inflammation due to the deposition of crystals either in the synovial fluid or in the soft tissue surrounding the joint. Polymorphs, attracted by chemotactic agents, phagocytose the crystals and attempt to digest the vast quantities of released kinines, lysosomal enzymes and other inflammatory substances. Crystal induced forms of inflammation are characterized by extremely severe pain and swelling which are much worse than those seen in chronic inflammatory arthritis. They may be confused with septic arthritis.

The principal forms of crystal induced inflammation are as follows:

1. Gout due to deposits of monosodium urate.
2. Pyrophosphate arthropathy due to calcium pyrophosphate crystals.
3. Post-intra-articular steroid injection due to the crystalline nature of the preparation.
4. Calcific periarthritis due to calcium hydroxyapatite crystals in the capsule and surrounding tissues.

Gout

Gout is more common in males in whom it starts in the third and fourth decades, whereas in women it usually starts after the menopause. Deposition of monosodium urate in the joint is usually but not always associated with elevated blood uric acid levels. In *primary gout* no cause for this can be identified. *Secondary gout* may be associated with increased formation of urate as in blood dyscrasias such as polycythaemia rubra vera, cytotoxic therapy of leukaemias and certain enzyme deficiencies and inhibition of urinary urate excretion which may be due to drugs such as thiazide diuretics or to renal impairment.

Acute gout is characterized by extremely severe inflammation most commonly in the metatarsophalangeal joint of the great toe but sometimes in the ankle, knee, small joints of the hands, wrists and elsewhere. The joint becomes extremely swollen and tender with erythema of the overlying skin. If untreated this severe pain and swelling may persist for several weeks before remitting. Recurrent attacks may occur with the joint relatively normal in between. However, in the course of time tophaceous deposits of monosodium urate disrupt and destroy the articular tissues producing deformities, disabilities and chronic pain. Tophi may also develop in the pinnae of the ears, over pressure points such as the elbows, in the kidneys producing renal damage, and elsewhere.

The management of acute and chronic gout are different. In acute gout high doses of anti-inflammatory drugs will usually produce remission of the inflammation within 24 or 48 hours. Indomethacin is extremely effective and may be given in a dose of 200 mg on the first day, 150 on the second day, 100 mg on the third and 100 mg from the third day onwards. Propionic acid derivatives such as naproxen may be used similarly. However aspirin is contraindicated in gout. In low doses it has uric acid retaining properties and may aggravate the underlying metabolic problem.

In patients with recurrent attacks of gout or with chronic tophaceous gout the decision must be made whether to embark on hypo-uricaemic therapy. Once started such treatment is generally maintained for life. However, one or two attacks of acute gout every couple of years can be managed with the use of anti-inflammatory drugs alone and long term hypouricaemic therapy is not indicated.

Uric acid formation is reduced by allopurinol usually given in a dose of 300 mg per day. Increased urinary urate excretion can be achieved by using probenicid 0.5 to 1.5 mg per day. Azapropazone has both anti-inflammatory and uricosuric properties and may have an advantage but it is more expensive. The uricosuric drugs are contraindicated if there is any evidence of renal damage because increased renal urate transport may exacerbate the problem. These drugs are so effective that failure to lower the blood uric level is more likely to be due to patient non-compliance than to any other cause. Side effects are uncommon but include gastrointestinal problems and hypersensitivity reactions.

During the first weeks of hypouricaemic therapy, mobilization of urate deposits can actually provoke an attack of gout which may be the most severe the patient has ever experienced. To prevent this the patient should receive prophylactic anti-inflammatory therapy usually with indomethacin or naproxen during the first two months of treatment.

Calcium pyrophosphate arthropathy

Deposition of calcium pyrophosphate dihydrate (CPPD) can provoke a variety of patterns of arthritis including extremely severe joint inflammation resembling gout ('pseudo-gout'), chronic inflammatory arthritis and osteroarthritis. However sometimes it may be a chance finding in a symptom free subject. It can be recognized by the presence of calcification of articular cartilage or knee menisci on radiographs and by demonstration of weakly positively birefringent crystals in synovial fluid. The underlying metabolic defect causing deposition of CPPD is usually not identified. This syndrome may occur in association with hyperparathyroidism, haemochromatosis, diabetes mellitus and other metabolic disorders.

Treatment is generally with non-steroidal anti-inflammatory drugs and the majority of cases will remit rapidly. Intra-articular injections of corticosteroids may also be indicated. Any metabolic disorder should be treated appropriately.

Calcific periarthritis

Calcium hydroxyapatite may be deposited in the soft tissues surrounding a joint provoking such severe inflammation that it may resemble acute arthritis. The most common site is the shoulder with involvement of the supraspinatus tendon. The range of movements is painful and restricted. X-rays show soft tissue calcification which is often transient, disappearing as the periarthritis remits.

This condition is treated with anti-inflammatory drugs and occasionally local steroid injections.

Osteoarthritis

Evidence of degenerative joint disease can be found in nearly all old people. Radiographs show a very high prevalence of osteoarthritic change. However, although it is common in the elderly, osteoarthritis seldom causes clinical problems.

Osteoarthritis may develop because of absolute or relative overuse of the joint. Occupational damage can lead to patterns of osteoarthritis in the hands in textile workers and in the knees of carpet layers and coal miners. Relative overuse may be a result of anatomical defects in joint structure due to developmental abnormalities, joint damage following trauma or inflammatory arthritis and various metabolic or endocrine diseases affecting the cartilage. Some patients show a pattern of generalized osteoarthritis particularly affecting distal inter-phalangeal (DIP) joints, the proximal interphalangeal (PIP) joints, the carpometacarpal joint of the thumb, the lumbar apophyseal joints and the first metatarsophalangeal (MTP) joint. This is known as primary generalized osteoarthritis and predominantly develops in post-menopausal females.

There is fibrillation, fasciculation and erosion of the articular cartilage. Microfractures occur in the underlying bone and heal leading to increased articular bone density–sclerosis. New bone formation at the margins of the joint (osteophytes) represents a reflex attempt to spread the articular load and restrict joint motion. Weakness and wasting of the muscles controlling the joint is common and may contribute towards instability. Pain does not arise from the articular cartilage, which does not contain nerve endings, but from the surrounding ligaments and tendons. These may be stretched or damaged causing trabecular microfractures within the sub-articular bone, increased vascular pressure within the epiphysis, secondary synovitis due to debris released within the joint and trapping of synovial fronds between the articular surfaces.

Pain is generally aggravated by physical activity and relieved by rest. After a night's sleep the patient may take a few seconds to get going but does not experience the prolonged morning stiffness that occurs in rheumatoid arthritis. The sensation of crepitus occurs during joint motion and joint movement may be restricted and deformity develop. The resultant loss of function leads to permanent disability.

Osteophytosis of the DIP joints and PIP joints leads to stiffness of the fingers but usually the patient is more worried by the appearance of the fingers and the fear of becoming permanently crippled. Appropriate reassurance may be all that is required. Involvement of the carpometa-carpal joint at the base of the thumb produces the appearance of squaring of the hand and pain on gripping any object. In the feet the common site of involvement is the first MTP joint which may develop a severe valgus deformity (bunion) with pressure of the medial osteophyte on the shoe producing severe pain when walking. In hallux rigidus the MTP joint is fixed in a neutral position and produces severe pain when walking because of the lack of flexion and extension movements. In the knee osteoarthritis may affect the medial or lateral tibio-femoral compartments or the patello-femoral joint. Severe pain may develop on walking and valgus, varus or flexion deformities develop. With hip disease the pain may be felt in the thigh and knee and not infrequently is mis-diagnosed as arising from the knee. The patient may develop a fixed deformity of flexion, adduction and external rotation. This may lead to apparent shortening of that lower limb and further difficulty in walking. When both hips are involved there may be major difficulties with personal hygiene.

Management of osteoarthritis

Management demands individual assessment of each patient and analysis of his particular problems. Anxiety or depression considerably exacerbate the perception of symptoms and appropriate reassurance or treatment is necessary.

Reducing the load on the damaged joint provides a lot of relief. Patients should be instructed to restrict exercise to that which does not produce pain and to regard the development of pain as a warning to do no more. All physical activities short of this should be encouraged. Resting painful joints in a splint may be helpful; a wrist splint will relieve thumb base arthritis yet allow virtually normal use of the hands. *Impulse loading* of joints should be avoided; for example the simple expedient of shock absorbing rubber heels to shoes may relieve pain in the hip or knee. A walking aid such as a stick will reduce the load on an osteoarthritic hip but care must be taken to ensure the stick is of the right length with a handle that the patient can grip adequately and that the patient knows how to use it properly. For unilateral osteoarthritis it should be held in the contralateral hand.

Physiotherapy techniques include pain relieving procedures such as ultrasonics, short wave diathermy, ice packs etc. and exercises which are aimed at strengthening the muscles and restoring and retaining joint function.

The non-steroidal anti-inflammatory drugs seem more effective than pure analgesics. The same drugs are used as in rheumatoid arthritis and the type of drug and the mode of administration are related to the patient's symptoms. For some the NSAIDs only provide partial relief and they may be supplemented by analgesics such as paracetamol, dextropropoxyphene or codeine.

In selected cases local steroid injections may be helpful. When the pain appears to arise from the surrounding ligaments and there is a localized tender area, pressure on which reproduces the symptoms, local infiltration with a long acting steroid may provide remarkable and prolonged relief. Some osteoarthritic joints develop acute flares of synovitis perhaps due to debris trapped between the articular surfaces. Intra-articular steroids may then be helpful. Strict asepsis is essential and these injections should only be performed by those with appropriate experience.

Surgery is indicated for advanced osteoarthritis. Excision arthroplasty is performed for hallux valgus relieving the pain directly from the damaged joint and from pressure on the bunion. Excision of the trapezium may relieve thumb base arthritis. Arthrodesis is now performed relatively rarely. Joint replacement operations are now very successful and total knee and hip replacements can produce enormous benefits for severe cases.

Back pain and sciatica

Back pain is a symptom with a large number of different causes (Table 2) and with varying forms of management. In communities with heavy emphasis on manual labour most back pains are of mechanical origin. Full assessment and investigation are necessary to differentiate these from other problems. There are a number of dynamic activities in which the back is involved. The patient bends, twists or lifts and develops acute pain and finds he is unable to straighten up. With a *prolapsed* disc this pain is initially felt in the lumbar region and may then radiate into the lower limb. The distribution of symptoms and physical signs is a guide to the particular nerve root that is involved. Acute episodes of pain usually last a few hours or in more severe cases a few days but they gradually wear off until the next bout occurs. The patient may identify specific movements, and in particular bending and lifting, that will produce pain. There may be a problem with chairs and prolonged sitting in a poor posture and a soft bed may aggravate the problem.

Table 2 Some causes of chronic back pain and sciatica

Recurrent low back strain
Facet syndrome
Abnormal articular facets
Osteophyte(s)
Osteomyelitis
Prolapsed intervertebral disc
Tuberculosis of the spine

Management of back pain of structural origin

Individual bouts of severe pain are usually of relatively limited duration. The patient makes a full or partial recovery until the next episode occurs. Treatment therefore requires relief of the acute episode, control of chronic symptoms and advice and help in an effort to prevent further episodes of pain.

In acute back pain with or without sciatica, bed rest is extremely important. Otherwise the pain will persist continuously or intermittently for long periods. Complete bed rest facilitates resolution within a few days or a couple of weeks. Complete bed rest means lying flat in bed with only one pillow on a properly supported mattress or firm surface. Soft beds sag readily and exacerbate back problems. A board under the mattress, which runs the full length of the bed and is at least as wide as the patient, is remarkably effective. Patients are allowed up only for toilet and washing.

As soon as the pain has remitted significantly, the patient is allowed to remobilize but must be careful to avoid stressing the back. He should lever himself up carefully using his arms, avoiding flexing the back and doing heavy lifting. In this acute stage a lumbo-sacral corset is useful and works by both splinting the spine and by increasing the intra-abdominal pressure. However it should only be used for a few weeks as prolonged use can lead to permanent stiffness of the back and further pain. Analgesic drugs are required. Non-steroidal anti-inflammatory drugs are usually more effective than other analgesics. Many patients develop severe aching and stiffness after a night's rest in bed and this is probably due to a secondary inflammation. Bed rest provides complete relief while the patient is at rest but pain develops on exercise, and analgesics such as dihydrocodeine and dextropropoxyphene are required. Narcotic analgesics should be avoided because of the risk of addiction in chronic back pain sufferers.

Detailed advice should be given to all patients to reduce the stress on the spine and prevent recurrences of back pain. Provision of instruction on care of the back is probably the most important role for the physiotherapist. The subject should stand upright with a flat lumbar spine, avoid lifting objects that are too heavy, carry weights close to the body and not at arm's length and not lift weights above the head. Lifting from the floor should be performed by standing with one foot behind and the other beside the object. The person who is lifting squats down with the object between his knees and the back straight or inclined forwards (see Figure 1). The object is firmly grasped with both hands and then lifted using the powerful hip and

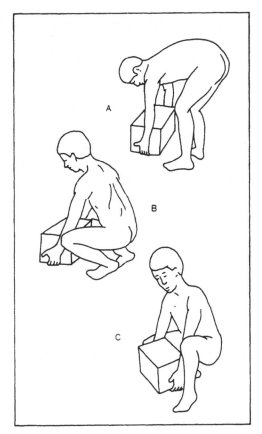

Figure 1 Methods of lifting. A: Wrong. B: Good. C: Best. Adapted from Jayson, M.I.V. (1983) (Oxford University Press), with permission from the author and publishers.

thigh muscles to straighten up. An upright chair with an adequate lumbar support or a small pillow in the lumbar area will relieve a lot of the problems associated with poor seating.

Exercises are often harmful particularly by mobilizing joints and ligaments that have already been damaged. Isometric exercises aimed at strengthening the paraspinal and abdominal muscles are beneficial. They stabilize the spine and increase the intra-abdominal pressure so relieving the spine of a proportion of its load. Traction, short-wave diathermy, ultrasonics, ice packs are effective at the time they are given but it is doubtful whether they have any lasting value.

Injection of local anaesthetic and steroids into painful and tender areas is sometimes helpful. Careful palpation of the back is required to identify the appropriate site and this technique is most likely to help when pressure on a single area reproduces the patient's symptoms.

Injections into the epidural space are given by the lumbar or the sacral route (see Chapter 13). They are most helpful for patients with sciatica which has not resolved following a period of complete bed rest.

There are few indications for surgery, which consists of laminectomy and decompression of nerve roots, removal of a damaged disc and fusion of vertebrae. Careful assessment and investigation of individual cases is required to decide which procedures are appropriate. The indications for operation are as follows:

1. Significant and unremitting symptoms despite an adequate period of conservative medical treatment including a period of supervised complete bed rest.
2. Persisting or advancing neurological signs. Of particular importance are cauda equina lesions with bladder or bowel involvement which may require emergency surgical decompression.
3. Recurrent attacks of severe pain and persistent disability such as the inability to perform normal work.

In general, surgery is more effective for sciatic pain than for back ache alone. As a rough guide 8 out of every 10 patients will be completely relieved of lower limb pain but only 5 or 6 relieved of back pain.

Soft tissue rheumatism

There are many patients with recurrent rheumatic symptoms (pain, aching and stiffness) in whom it is difficult to make a specific diagnosis. The aches and pains may be generalized or limited to the neck, back or parts of the limbs. Periodic individual assessment is necessary because the underlying diagnosis may only become apparent during long term follow up.

General aches and pains

Aches and pains may be prodromal features of rheumatoid arthritis or other forms of inflammatory joints disease. *Polymyalgia rheumatica* usually affects elderly people, more often females, with complaints of aching and stiffness around the limb girdles and may be complicated by temporal, retinal or cranial arteritis. In general the ESR is very high. Treatment with steroids is usually dramatically successful.

Metabolic bone disease, and particularly hypo- and hypercalcaemia and widespread Paget's disease, can produce generalized bone pain and aching with acute exacerbations if fractures occur. Malignancy can present as ill health and generalized aches and pains. Hypothyroidism and hyperthyroidism can also present in this way. Certain patients taking the contraceptive pill or barbiturates develop aches and pains particularly in the limbs.

Local pain syndromes

Pain in and around the *shoulder* is remarkably common. Careful examination will determine whether the pain actually arises in the shoulder or is referred from the neck or the viscera. Localized disorders include not only bone and joint disease but also soft tissue lesions such as supraspinatus tendinitis, bicipital tendinitis, rotator cuff lesions and frozen shoulders. Some patients have extremely tender focal areas usually over the scapulae. These localized problems will usually respond to an accurately placed local steroid injection or to physiotherapy treatment as appropriate.

Pain in the *elbow* may be referred from the neck or be due to bone and joint disease. Very common are lateral *epicondylitis* and medial epicondylitis. The elbow movements appear full but the symptoms are reproduced by pressure over the lateral and medial epicondyles respectively. They usually respond to local steroid injection or physiotherapy treatment.

In the *hands* pain can be due to a wide variety of bone, joint, tendon, vascular and local or referred neurological problems. *Tenosynovitis* can affect the dorsal or palmar tendons producing pain, stiffness and difficulty in using the fingers. Involvement of the extensor tendon of the thumb may occur in people who do repeated thumb movements. On occasions tenosynovitis can be the presenting feature of inflammatory arthritis. Tenosynovitis will usually respond to rest, physiotherapy and sometimes local steroid injections. The injection may be given into the tendon sheath, but not into the substance of the tendon itself as it may produce necrosis and tendon rupture.

In the *carpal tunnel syndrome*, median nerve compression produces pain and paraesthesiae in the fingers which are poorly localized to the median nerve distribution and often radiate proximally up the whole of the upper limb even as far as the neck. It is characteristic that these symptoms occur during the night waking the patient, who obtains relief by hanging the hand out of bed and flexing and extending the fingers. There may be motor and sensory signs of median nerve damage and the diagnosis is confirmed by nerve conduction studies. This condition may occur on its own but may be a presenting feature of weight gain, inflammatory arthritis, hypothyroidism or other disorders. The underlying condition should be treated and in particular weight loss may relieve the problem. Resting the hand in a splint in a neutral position at night may help. Injection of a long-acting steroid through the flexor retinaculum into the carpal tunnel avoiding the median nerve is usually effective. Median nerve decompression may be necessary for more severe cases particularly if there is wasting of the muscles of the thenar eminence.

A multitude of problems produce *pain in the feet*. These include not only bone, joint and soft tissue disorders but also vascular disorders and referred pain from more proximal lesions.

Metatarsalgia is pain in the forefoot usually relieved by applying padding under the metatarsal heads. Specific problems such as Morton's neurofibroma and march fractures should be identified. In the hindfoot pain may occur under the heel (plantar fasciitis) or behind the heel (Achilles' tendinitis). Relief from pressure, physiotherapy treatment and occasionally careful local steroid injections (not into the tendon itself) are helpful.

Pain felt in the knee may be due to arthritis but also meniscal and ligamentous lesions, bone disorders, pre-patella and infra-patella bursitis, popliteal cysts or be referred from the hip, spine or pelvis. Soft tissue problems around the knee can be treated by relief from stress, physiotherapy or local steroid injections.

Pain is felt in the hip for many reasons apart from various forms of arthritis affecting the joint. In trochanteric bursitis pain which can be severe is felt in the lateral aspect of the hip. Examination shows a full range of hip movements but extreme focal tenderness over the greater trochanter. This usually responds to physiotherapy or local injection of steroid.

Recommended reading

Jayson, M.I.V. (1980). *The Lumbar Spine and Back Pain.* (London: Pitman Medical)
Jayson, M.I.V. and Million, R. (1983). *Locomotor Disability in General Practice.* (Oxford University Press)
Scott, J.T. (1978). *Copeman's Textbook of Rheumatic Diseases.* (Edinburgh: Churchill Livingstone)

9

Vascular Disease

Sydney Rose

Introduction

This chapter deals with chronic pain resulting from diseases of the peripheral vascular system.

Table 1 shows a classification of vascular conditions which give rise to pain.

Table 1

I. Chronic pain of arterial origin

A. *Main arteries*
    i. Occlusive disease
    ii. Aneurysm
    iii. Embolism

B. *Peripheral arteries*
    i. Buerger's disease (thrombo-angiitis obliterans)
    ii. Diabetic arteritis
    iii. Arteritis associated with collagen diseases
    iv. The role of vasospasm
    v. Miscellaneous conditions
       Erythromelalgia, trench foot, immersion foot, frostbite and others.

II. Chronic pain of venous origin

A. *Venous incompetence*
    i. Superficial venous incompetence
    ii. Deep venous incompetence

B. *Phlebitis*
    i. Superficial
    ii. Deep

Clinical examination

A patient with a suspected vascular disorder requires a careful history, which includes mode of onset, duration, progress of the symptoms, past medical records and the social and family history. Current medications and smoking habits should be recorded. The general appearance of the patient should be assessed noting obvious abnormalities such as gross obesity, wasting, anaemia, and the age/appearance relationship. The patient should be seen standing and walking with special reference to abnormalities of gait. It should be noted if he is in obvious pain.

Next a routine examination of the heart and lungs should be carried out and the blood pressure taken in both arms. The abdomen should be examined in a routine fashion but particular attention is given to identifying the presence of an abnormal mass especially if pulsatile. If this is found, an attempt should be made to decide whether the pulsation is expansile or transmitted. Examination in the knee-elbow position will usually help to make this distinction. The presence of enlarged veins running from groin to costal margin should be noted as they may be an indication of inferior vena cava block. Every abdominal examination must be completed by a rectal examination. Any prostatic enlargement must be noted, for otherwise acute retention may be an unexpected complication if surgery is necessary.

Examination of the pulses

The carotid pulses must be carefully examined by palpation and auscultation. Any inequality or the presence of bruits must be noted. The radial pulse will not only give information about any cardiac irregularity or occlusion in the upper limb but will enable the state of the arterial wall to be estimated. The femoral pulses should also be examined by palpation and auscultation. Dilatation or calcification will be noted as well as an inequality or the presence of a conducted bruit.

Marked reduction of pulsation in one or both legs indicates aorto-iliac occlusion or stenosis. The pulses should be traced down the thigh as far as possible. The popliteal pulses are best palpated with the patient in the prone position with the knee slightly flexed.

The posterior tibial pulse is consistently placed and is located halfway between the internal malleolus and the edge of the heel. The dorsalis pedis pulse is usually found at or near to the midline at the front of the ankle joint but if it divides into its medial and lateral branches at a higher level it may seem to be absent.

Examination of the pulses must be followed by a survey of the hips, knees, ankle and shoulder joints, the cervical and lumbosacral spine and in particular the presence of limitation of straight leg raising and the condition of the peripheral reflexes. Many of the pains that are thought to be of vascular origin arise in the skeletal system.

Evidence of muscle wasting in the limbs should be noted and the nutritional condition of the skin of the feet and hands should be assessed. Loss of hair distally in the lower limbs, cracking of the nails, and atrophy of toe pads indicate diminution of peripheral circulation while marked colour changes in the toes and feet on elevation and dependency may be present. Cyanosis of the toes and cold feet alone in the presence of a peripheral pulse merely indicate vasospasm and may indeed be normal in some individuals. On the other hand painful red shiny toes of recent onset with absent pulses suggest severe arterial insufficiency. Examination of the retinal vessels by ophthalmoscopy will give direct evidence of arteriosclerosis or of diabetic retinopathy.

The use of an oscillometer (Pachon, Von Recklinghausen or Collins) can be helpful especially in comparing the circulation in both limbs and there is a simple and inexpensive Doppler (Sonicaid) to detect peripheral blood flow.

DISEASE OF MAIN ARTERIES

Occlusive arterial disease

This gives rise to the pain of intermittent claudication, ischaemic rest pain, and the pain of ischaemic ulceration and gangrene. No single factor has been identified as a specific cause of occlusive arterial disease. Heredity, race, social circumstance, age, sex, diet, smoking, diabetes mellitus, haemodynamic wear and tear, all have an influence on the origin and progress of the disease. The ratio of males to females is almost three to one, but the condition is rare in women before the menopause. Thereafter the incidence of arteriosclerosis becomes increasingly common. After the age of 65 the disease affects both sexes equally.

The signs and symptoms of arterial occlusive disease are due to impaired blood supply to the limb distal to the occlusion. This may be in the aortic arch, the subclavian vessels, the aortoiliac segment, the femoropopliteal vessels or the peripheral arteries themselves. The condition will be asymptomatic until the degree of narrowing is sufficient to alter the peripheral blood flow. Much depends on the demand for oxygenated blood and symptoms will develop much earlier in a young and active man in full employment than in an elderly retired patient, perhaps already slowed down by arthritis, heart disease or chronic bronchitis.

Chronic intermittent claudication

In a patient with occlusive arterial disease removal of accumulated metabolites from the muscles is inadequate during exercise; when the patient rests the arterial supply catches up and the metabolites are cleared. This produces spasmodic cramp-like pain – the so-called *intermittent claudication*. It occurs most frequently in the calf muscle because stenosis commonly occurs in the femoropopliteal vessels. The sensation of tightness or pain usually starts at the same 'trigger' point on each occasion and may radiate up or down the leg.

These symptoms are exacerbated by exercise and may be intensified or reproduced by firm digital pressure over the calf muscle (Figure 1).

The pain of intermittent claudication is at first a slight tightness in the affected muscle, which may pass off as exercise (which normally produces vasodilatation) continues. As the condition progresses there develops a definite though tolerable pain as walking continues, which

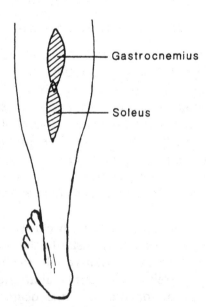

Gastrocnemius

Soleus

Figure 1　Claudication pressure points

can become so intense that the patient has to stop in 50 yards or less. Intermittent claudication is graded into 3 categories (Figure 2):

1. The tightness in the affected muscle passes off with walking

2. The pain stabilizes with exercise and the patient may go for a considerable further distance before needing to stop

3. The pain is severe, comes on quickly and brings the patient to an immediate halt.

When the patient has rested for a minute or two he will often continue for the same distance again before being brought to a halt once more. If he walks more quickly, or uphill, or against the wind, he will be brought to a halt sooner. The cardinal diagnostic point in intermittent claudication is the definite and consistent relationship to exercise, and this fact distinguishes it from all other pains. The intensity of symptoms varies with the extent of the disease. The average patient shows a steady decline in performance over a period of time. This deterioration is often steplike rather than continuous and depends on the development of collateral circulation which may for a time compensate for the diminished peripheral flow (Figure 3).

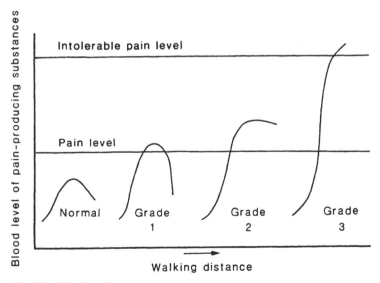

Figure 2   Claudication diagram

In contrast to this close relationship to exercise is a condition known as *pseudo-claudication* which may occur in patients with an atypical sciatica. The presence of good peripheral pulses should serve to differentiate this condition while straight leg raising will be limited and produce pain at the back of the thigh. Occasionally osteoarthritis of the hip, knee or ankle can simulate claudication but careful history taking and detailed clinical examination should identify pain related to a stiff and creaking joint.

Pain in the calf may also be due to varicose veins or old deep venous thrombosis but this pain is always relieved by elevation of the limb and is often relieved rather than aggravated by exercise. However, these conditions may co-exist with peripheral arterial disease.

Claudication in the forearm is much less frequent because of the different type of activity of the upper limb. It may appear in patients whose work involves intricate repetitive hand movements. The symptoms may be especially apparent when exercise combined with elevation of the arm is involved – for example a woman hanging out clothes, or alternatively carrying out the repeated arm movements of ironing, washing or polishing. Occlusion of arteriosclerotic vessels can be precipitated by trauma.

Ischaemic rest pain

Pain develops when arterial occlusion is advanced; when tissue perfusion slows to a halt gangrene occurs.

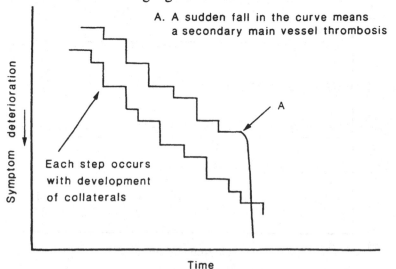

Figure 3   Deterioration of the arterial perfusion with time

The skin can tolerate a low blood supply much better than sensory nerve end organs and therefore pain is experienced in the ischaemic nerve long before ulceration occurs. Pain in the toes and across the metatarsal heads is usually gradual in onset and troublesome mainly at night. During sleep there is a generalized vasodilatation and blood drains away from the toes into the heel. Intense pain wakes the patient who obtains relief by getting up and walking about. Ultimately he finds that he can get respite by hanging the leg out of bed or putting it on a pillow on a low chair by the side of the bed; this maintains the blood supply to the toes mainly by gravity but has the disadvantage of producing oedema. As the condition progresses rest pain becomes constant, severe and requires increasingly powerful analgesics. The toes become red and shiny with loss of pulp, the nails cracked and dry, localized areas of skin necrosis appear.

Ischaemic rest pain may occur suddenly without any preceding history of intermittent claudication, or with claudication so mild as to escape attention. Usually however, it is the ultimate expression of a gradual increase of ischaemia with dwindling claudication distance becoming progressively apparent. Ischaemic pain is due to accumulation of toxic metabolites.

Peripheral neuritis due to diabetes can simulate rest pain but peripheral pulses are palpable and the symptoms often respond to antidiabetic therapy and large doses of vitamin B12 (1 ampoule i.m. alternate days for two weeks followed by cyanocobalamin 100 micrograms b.d. orally for four weeks). In the later stages there is diminished or absent sensation when the nerve ends have atrophied.

Popliteal entrapment syndrome

This is an uncommon but interesting variety of intermittent claudication which occurs in young, fit and athletic individuals. It is caused by intermittent compression of the popliteal artery under the two heads of a well-developed gastrocnemius muscle or under the soleal arch. Claudication symptoms only occur during severe physical exertion.

Clinical examination is rarely helpful and the condition is only diagnosed by peripheral arteriography. If arteriography is not available, the measurement of the brachial and ankle pulse pressure before and immediately after exercise may substantiate the diagnosis. The normal ratio is 1 but it may reduce to 0.5 to 0.7 after exercise and then return to normal after a period of rest. If it is abnormal at rest, then some degree of occlusion should be suspected.

If there is still clinical doubt and arteriography is not available the patient should be referred to the nearest cardiovascular centre.

Laboratory investigations for arterial disease

1. *Serum electrolytes.* Sodium, potassium, chloride, alkali reserve, creatinine and urea levels to eliminate acidosis, alkalosis or impaired renal function.
2. *Resting glucose tolerance* to test for overt or subclinical diabetes.
3. *Serum lipids* are estimated including fasting cholesterol, triglycerides and lipoprotein levels. Raised cholesterol and in particular triglycerides are risk factors in arteriosclerosis.
4. *A full blood count* and differential white cell count to reveal anaemia or more particularly polycythaemia which can be a cause of intravascular clotting.

If these tests are difficult to obtain the most important are the glucose tolerance test and the blood count. In addition to these blood tests the urine should be tested for sugar, blood and albumin.

Treatment of occlusive arterial disease

The treatment of pain due to occlusive arterial disease may be conservative or operative. Many vascular surgeons believe that surgery is the only effective treatment but conservative treatment must not be ignored.

The decision on the method of treatment of intermittent claudication depends on the severity of the symptoms and the exercise needs of the individual. It must also relate to his age and general condition.

Conservative (non-operative) management

a. *Intermittent claudication*

In minor cases continued observation is all that is necessary. Vasodilator drugs may be helpful if there is an element of vasospasm (see page 103). Their use involves continuous observation of the patient's progress. Patients must be persuaded to give up smoking cigarettes.

b. *Ischaemic rest pain and gangrene*

1. Eliminate sepsis by the use of appropriate antibiotics.

2. Removal of dead tissue to allow drainage of pus and to promote healing. This can often be done without general anaesthesia under analgesic sedation.

3. Dressings should be soaked in hypertonic saline followed by half strength Eusol (sodium hypochlorate). Irrigation of infected pockets with 3% hydrogen peroxide in diabetic gangrene is extremely valuable in relief of pain, especially when there is an anaerobic infection. Another useful preparation is a dressing of urea peroxide in glycerine which releases oxygen in the depths of the ulcer and removes the dead tissue. The composition of the preparations is given on page 118.

4. Protect the limb from exposure to extremes of temperature and trauma. A padded bed cage is useful to protect the feet. The patient is often more comfortable sleeping with the limb somewhat dependent and this is achieved by raising the head end of the bed on 13 cm blocks.

6. Analgesic drugs (see Chapter 12). However, many patients with diabetic gangrene are often surprisingly pain-free because peripheral neuritis causes loss of sensation.

Vasodilator therapy

It is unreasonable to expect that a vasodilator drug can effectively dilate a sclerotic vessel. However the object of their use is to dilate the collateral vessels and other peripheral vessels which are not involved in the disease. Also vasodilators may regulate the increase in vasomotor tone which is often present. Many people living in damp and cool climates are subject to mild vasospastic disorders as a constitutional defect, and they complain of cold hands and feet even in mild weather. These symptoms will be aggravated if the patient develops arteriosclerosis.

The site and mode of action of vasodilator drugs varies considerably and the response varies in different individuals. The treatment therefore must be regulated according to the response.

The most potent vasodilator available is tolazolene which is rather expensive. Many patients are unable to tolerate it because of gastrointestinal and other side effects which may occur before the vasodilator effect is established. It should be avoided in patients with a history of indigestion. The initial dose is 25 mg twice a day increasing to 50 mg three or four times a day when tolerance is established.

Other drugs are selected by clinical trial or by comparative digital plethysmography if this facility is available. The drugs recommended are bamethan sulphate 25 mg 4 times daily and nicotinyl tartrate 25 mg one or two tablets 4 times daily.

Other conservative measures

Another technique practised in some countries is that of intra-arterial perfusion. This may be carried out either by daily puncture of the femoral artery until improvement occurs (not more than ten days in all) or by continuous infusion most economically achieved by using an indwelling arterial catheter and a Fenwall bag containing the perfusion fluid and inflated to a pressure of 300 mm of mercury. This drips through an ordinary intravenous drip chamber. The principle is one of arterial bouginage using a solution containing a vasodilator, heparin, an antibiotic and a low molecular dextran base to improve tissue perfusion. The pack may simply be incorporated into a sphygmomanometer cuff if a Fenwall bag is not available. One litre of fluid is given every 16 hours for three days.

Intra-arterial bouginage (see Recommended Reading)

Another non-operative technique to overcome arterial stenosis or occlusion is that of percutaneous intra-arterial bouginage with balloon catheters. A balloon catheter is passed up or down the affected artery and the stenosed area dilated under X-ray control. If this technique fails however arterial surgery should be available immediately.

For details of perfusion solution see p. 118.

Direct arterial surgery

Direct arterial surgery is the treatment of choice in arterial occlusion. The symptoms must have been established for at least six months to allow natural recovery to occur by development of the collateral circulation. When the condition has stabilized and the symptoms warrant it surgical treatment must be considered.

If however claudication has proceeded to the stage where pain comes on after walking as little as 50 yards or less, the onset of constant rest pain is imminent and the problem becomes more acute. It is then not so much a problem of treating claudication as of limb salvage. Direct arterial surgery is justified but it should not be undertaken unless arteriographic facilities and blood transfusion are available and the surgeon has had sufficient training.

The details of the technique of direct arterial surgery are beyond the scope of the present chapter. The by-pass procedure can restore the blood flow to normal and is the treatment of choice whenever feasible (see Recommended Reading).

In those patients who are unfit for direct arterial surgery or for whom these procedures are not available for one reason or another, lumbar sympathectomy is a possible palliative alternative for rest pain where gangrene is not yet established.

Lumbar sympathectomy

Lumbar sympathectomy may improve the blood supply to the skin at the periphery and preserve skin cover, thus averting gangrene. In addition it is often successful in relieving rest pain and incipient or even established gangrene of the toes, especially when this is limited to the second, third and fourth toes. The most difficult areas to heal are the big toe, the dorsum of the foot and the heel. The earlier surgery is performed the higher the success rate.

There is no doubt that if cases are carefully selected for sympathectomy, and this applies to both chemical and surgical sympathectomy, good results can be obtained. It will help in intermittent claudication where there is a good collateral circulation. With gangrene it is of most value in limiting the extent of skin necrosis by producing a clear line of demarcation.

Lumbar sympathectomy can be achieved surgically, by removing the sympathetic chain (see Recommended Reading) or chemically by percutaneous neurolytic injection of the ganglia.

Sympathetic block

An alternative technique to improve peripheral circulation is a paravertebral sympathetic block with 5–10% aqueous phenol which is recommended in aged patients or in those considered to be too ill to undergo surgery. The technique is described in Chapter 13. It has been suggested that a prognostic paravertebral block should be carried out before surgical sympathectomy is undertaken but although a positive response is helpful, improvement is often seen even after a negative result.

In the elderly every effort should be made to preserve the limb; to render the patient immobile is a virtual death sentence. Nevertheless when all attempts to restore circulation have failed amputation must be considered before the patient becomes toxic and exhausted from pain and lack of sleep.

Aneurysms

Aneurysms may be arteriosclerotic or traumatic. They are slow to develop and do not give rise to much pain until they leak and perforate. They occasionally present with chronic aching pain associated with a swelling which gradually increases in size.

Traumatic aneurysms sometimes develop after a closed injury or a penetrating wound. They may also arise at a suture line after direct arterial surgery. Occasionally a communication develops between an artery and a vein following trauma resulting in an arteriovenous fistula. (For further details see Recommended Reading.)

PERIPHERAL ARTERIES

Buerger's disease (thromboangiitis obliterans)

This is an 'inflammatory' lesion of unknown aetiology affecting the vessels at arteriolar level in the early stages. Ninety to ninety-five per cent of the patients are men and the usual age of onset is between 20 and 40 years. The condition is rare in pure blooded Negroes. Most of the arterial disease which occurs in the Indian Subcontinent and the Far East is similar to thromboangiitis obliterans. Cigarette smoking is significantly related to the disease although the mechanism of its influence is not known. If cigarette smoking is discontinued spontaneous improvement will occur, and conversely a relapse will occur when cigarette smoking is resumed.

Pathology

The small arteries of the hands (30%) and feet (70%) are usually affected. Very rarely the hands are involved alone. The larger arteries of the limbs become involved at a later stage in direct contrast to arteriosclerosis. Occlusion of the arteries proximal to the wrist is rare, but the visceral arteries are sometimes involved. In 40% or more cases, a migrating superficial phlebitis is present at some time during the course of the condition usually in the early stages of the disease.

The typical pathological feature of Buerger's disease is an inflammatory process. The affected artery is surrounded by dense fibrosis, often involving the adjacent vein, and occasionally a concomitant nerve too. This contrasts with the arteriosclerotic artery which does not become adherent to the vein unless it is calcified. Histologically the small thrombosed artery shows extensive proliferation of endothelial cells and fibroblasts. The wall of the artery is thickened, and the lumen narrowed but the overall architecture remains clear. Arterial occlusion is commonly segmental and extension of the disease is episodic in character, with quiescent periods during which collateral circulation develops and some recanalization occurs.

Symptoms and signs

Pain occurs either as claudication in the foot muscles, or as rest pain in the toes and forefoot, progressing to painful ulceration and gangrene after a variable interval of time. The onset is gradual, and usually starts with continuous severe burning pain and discolouration of a toe, the great toe being often involved. Usually one limb is affected but the second leg often becomes involved later, the interval between the two varying from months to years. Swelling and redness may be present in all the toes, which later become cyanosed. The venous return on pressure remains brisk because of the development of peripheral vasodilation. Dilated capillaries and dilated arterioles tend to give a warm red toe at first but as the venules dilate cyanosis develops.

The posterior tibial and dorsalis pedis pulses become obliterated at an early stage of the disease, but the popliteal pulse is not initially affected. Bilateral absent posterial tibial pulses are highly suggestive of Buerger's disease. The chronic ischaemia results in atrophy of the skin, loss of hair, brittle nails, and in more advanced cases, ulceration and gangrene of the digits, eventually extending onto the dorsum of the foot. In the upper limb gangrene may occur in the finger tips, but rarely spreads proximally.

Treatment

Cigarette smoking must be stopped immediately, no matter how difficult this may be.

Local measures: Infection should be treated by appropriate antibiotic therapy, and either local cleansing with lukewarm hypertonic saline solution or a local dressing of half-strength Eusol solution is applied over non-stick gauze. The feet must be protected from trauma, extremes of temperature and damp. Tight shoes must be avoided.

General measures:

1. Raise the head end of the bed by about 10 cm.

2. Oral anticoagulants should be started at once (phenindione 200 mg immediately followed by 50–100 mg daily according to prothrombin activity) while heparin is given i.v. for five days until the prothrombin value reaches the therapeutic level. Calcium heparin 5000 units s.c. 8 hourly for 5 days may be used.

3. Steroids are of value in the acute phase. Prednisolone 10 mg 4 times daily is recommended initially, reducing to 5 mg twice daily as soon as the inflammatory reaction is under control.

4. An intravenous infusion of low molecular weight dextran (dextran 70) is given to prevent peripheral 'sludging' of red cells and platelets, and thereby minimize or prevent gangrene by improving tissue perfusion. One unit is given daily for five days in the first instance and a second similar course can be given after a three day interval.

5. Vasodilator drugs are most indicated in those cases in which there is a history or evidence of vasospasm.

6. Surgical treatment. The only surgical treatment of value is lumbar sympathectomy with excision of the second, third and fourth lumbar ganglia or stellate ganglionectomy for the upper limb. Sympathectomy will only be indicated in cases which do not respond to conservative measures. In patients unfit or unwilling to undergo surgical sympathectomy, a chemical sympathetic block with phenol or alcohol is worthwhile. The condition may relapse however after periods varying from months to years, especially if the patient continues to smoke.

If amputation becomes necessary it should be as conservative as possible. A trans-metatarsal or Syme's operation must be considered first. A below knee amputation may be required before a soundly healed stump is achieved but this should be the last resort.

Diabetic arteritis

The effect of diabetes mellitus on the state of the arteries is often misunderstood. It may be: (1) the true diabetic (usually in the younger age group) who has established diabetes for many years before arterial symptoms develop; (2) the elderly arteriosclerotic patient in whom diabetes is a secondary manifestation of diminished blood supply to the islet cells of the pancreas and in whom, therefore, the symptoms of arterial insufficiency fall into the arteriosclerotic pattern.

In the true diabetic group, peripheral ulceration is caused by a combination of hypoaesthesia of the pressure areas of the foot due to peripheral neuritis and the development of sepsis under a callosity which, as it is prevented from discharging, causes spreading subcutaneous tissue necrosis with surprisingly little pain.

This localized gangrene is due more to sepsis than to peripheral vascular occlusion although a secondary diffuse non-specific obliterative arteritis is present. The necrotic tissue, however extensive, will separate and the lesion heal if the diabetic state is corrected.

Arteriosclerotic gangrene, by contrast, is always severely painful in the early stages, the pain being most severe when the limb is horizontal as in bed at night. The patient finds relief by allowing the limb to hang out of bed or by sitting up in a chair. When a clear line of demarcation develops between living and dead tissue the pain tends to abate.

Arteritis associated with collagen diseases

There are a number of collagen diseases with occlusion of the large and small arteries. Whether they are different diseases or different manifestations of the same condition is not yet resolved. Non-specific small vessel inflammatory response occurs in polyarteritis nodosa, diffuse lupus erythematosus, scleroderma, dermatomyositis, temporal arteritis and in 'nodular vasculitis'. In all these conditions there is a hyaline degeneration of the medial coat of the small arteries with proliferation of the intima. There is perivascular round cell infiltration with oedema and ultimate fibrosis.

This vascular condition is also found as a complication of rheumatoid arthritis. Pain in these cases is burning in nature and localized to the anatomical areas involved and responds rapidly to steroid therapy.

Raynaud's disease

This is a disturbance in the peripheral circulation associated with colour changes caused by exposure to cold or emotion. The condition is a symptom complex which is either primary idiopathic or secondary to occlusive vascular disease. It can become so severe that necrotic changes in the digital skin with severe chronic burning pain may develop without any evidence of occlusion of the major limb arteries. There is evidence to suggest that there is a local fault in the muscle wall of the digital arteries. The upper limb is the most affected. Response to cervico-thoracic sympathectomy is variable and recurrence of symptoms which often occurs may be explained by vaso 'spasm' which is not mediated through the cervicodorsal sympathetic chain.

Raynaud's disease is five times more common in women than in men, and arises before the fortieth year in 90% of cases. It occurs ten times more frequently in the upper limb than the lower and it is usually bilateral although one hand may be worse than the other. It is basically a disease of damp temperate climates.

Pathology

Colour changes in the skin depend on the capillary tone whereas temperature changes are related to the condition of the arterioles. In a typical attack, both the capillaries and arterioles go into spasm, giving rise to cold white fingers. The subsequent anoxia causes loss of tone in the capillary walls resulting in capillary vasodilatation. The blood flow stagnates in the dilated capillaries, the blood becomes increasingly deoxygenated and the fingers appear cold and cyanosed. Increasing anoxia produces paralysis of the arteriolar walls which relax and a flush appears, first causing a reddish blue colour in the skin and finally profound hyperaemia with red and slightly swollen fingers.

Treatment

Vasodilators are recommended only in mild cases. The patient is advised to keep warm. When exposed to cold, two layers of gloves should be advised. A thin pair of silk gloves under a pair of woollen gloves affords the best protection. The condition produces discomfort rather than pain but analgesics may be necessary, especially when the affected fingers are recovering. In more advanced cases cervico-dorsal sympathectomy is beneficial although the improvement is not as long lasting as that achieved by lumbar sympathectomy in cases with foot involvement.

Thoracic outlet syndrome

This involves the lower trunk of the brachial plexus (C8-T1 roots) and is due to compression of the nerves by fibrous bands, muscle or bone in the case of a cervical rib.

Pain may be referred to the shoulder, arm or localized areas of sensory distribution with occasional hypoaesthesia or localized muscle weakness. Secondary Raynaud symptoms develop when there is compression of the axillary artery as it crosses the first rib. In such cases downward and backward traction on the arm will obliterate the radial pulse.

Treatment is by identification of the underlying lesion and by surgical relief if the symptoms warrant it.

Collagen disorders

Scleroderma

This disorder involves the skin of the face, the lower oesophagus and the hands and wrists but may be confined to the periphery in some cases for many years. Raynaud's phenomenon in the hands may be one of the earliest symptoms. When this condition is advanced subcutaneous nodules (hypodermolithiasis) may occur in the pulps of the fingers. These nodules may eventually ulcerate and discharge calcareous material. This is a severely painful process. Healing will not occur until all the calcified material has been extruded. X-ray of the affected digit will show the area of calcification.

Treatment

Powerful analgesics may be required until permanent relief is obtained by curettage of the affected areas under general anaesthesia with removal of as much of the calcified material as possible.

Erythromelalgia

This condition consists of a burning, red, painful extremity with increased local skin temperature. The condition may be primary or secondary. The primary condition occurs in healthy individuals who have no detectable organic disease of the nervous or vascular systems. Little is known of the pathology and aetiology.

Secondary erythromelalgia is usually a symptom of vascular disease.

It occurs occasionally with hypertension and often with polycythaemia. It may also occur in cases of organic neurological disease,
poisoning by heavy metals, and in gout.

Pathophysiology

The raised skin temperature is the most important feature of the
syndrome. The temperature at which distress occurs varies in different
parts of the limb and usually ranges from 32°C to 36°C. When it rises
above the 'critical point' distressing pain occurs and may persist.
Burning pain can be initiated by warming the skin of the affected
limb or by lowering the limb. Raising the limb reduces the pain which
may also be relieved by direct local pressure on the affected area.

The presence of vasodilatation is shown by the increased skin
temperature, the increased amplitude of arterial pulsation, by a
throbbing sensation, by increased radiation of heat and by increased
oxygen content of the venous blood.

The condition occurs in both men and women, usually arising in
middle age or later. It is rare in children. Usually both hands and feet
are involved, but burning pain is often localized to a part of the foot.
The pain may come on during exercise or when the patient gets warm
in bed. The burning may last from a few minutes to several hours.
Distress is worse during warm weather.

The patient complains that the burning parts are reddish blue in
colour and that the skin is hot to touch. Trophic changes are unusual
in idiopathic cases but may occur in secondary erythromelalgia. The
affected parts may be locally oedematous and the whole limb may be
slightly swollen. In idiopathic cases there is no evidence of occlusive
arterial disease.

Treatment

Acetylsalicylic acid in divided doses for several days may produce
appreciable relief. The condition is improved by avoiding warmth,
and by the use of cold towels or cold packs at night. Phenoxybenzamine
10 mg twice daily or 3 times daily is often effective in bringing about
some improvement. In secondary erythromelalgia the underlying
condition should be treated.

Prognosis

In the idiopathic condition the episodes of distress continue indefinitely but there is no permanent disability. In the secondary condition the syndrome bears the prognosis of the underlying disease.

Trench foot and immersion foot

Peripheral circulatory changes result from exposure to damp and low temperatures but freezing of tissues does not occur. Lack of activity increases the effect. Immersion foot is a similar condition resulting from prolonged immersion of the feet in cold water. It is aggravated by standing and immobility of the legs and sometimes vitamin deficiency is an additional factor.

In immersion foot and trench foot, three phases are recognized:

1. *Early ischaemic stage*

   This stage persists as long as the leg is exposed or immersed. There is vaso-constriction of superficial arterioles and the extremities are pale or cyanosed and cold, with reduced or absent arterial pulsations. Orthostatic oedema will appear.

2. *Hyperaemic stage*

   When the patient has been moved to a warmer environment, the foot becomes red and hot with bounding pulses and swelling develops. This will increase unless the feet are raised and kept cool. Thrombosed small veins and scattered ecchymoses appear on the affected parts in the hyperaemic stage which may last from a few days to a few weeks and then subsides for no obvious reason. Ulceration and gangrene may develop in severe cases but is comparatively painless compared to the burning discomfort experienced in the limb prior to the development of skin necrosis which is usually quite superficial.

3. *Late ischaemic stage*

   In severe cases there is a very slow recovery with coldness, stiffness, pain and paraesthesia in the lower limbs, which are cold and blue even when the patient is warm. A secondary Raynaud's phenomenon is often present.

Treatment

1. The limbs should be kept cool at first but must be completely

dry. They must be protected from further trauma and wrapped in sterile towels to avoid infection. Parenteral and local antibiotics should be given to reduce inflammatory oedema and the patient kept in bed with warmth applied to the body. Gentle exercise should be instituted as soon as sensation returns. At a later stage local massage and mild heat should be given in the form of warm foot baths in non-ulcerated cases.

2. Drug therapy.

    The non-steroid anti-inflammatory drugs seem to have the greatest chance of success. Naproxen 500 mg twice daily for five days followed by 250 mg for the next five days usually brings about an immediate improvement. Indomethacin has also been used effectively.

3. If ulceration occurs or persists sympathetic ganglion blocking drugs are given or lumbar sympathetic block is carried out. The block may be repeated if necessary. Continuing disability is an indication for lumbar sympathectomy.

Frostbite

Acute frostbite leads to intense vasoconstriction, pallor and loss of sensation. If the cold and ischaemia are not quickly relieved, thrombosis of smaller arteries may produce death of tissues and gangrene. In mild frostbite the outer layers of the skin only are affected; in severe frostbite the deeper tissues are involved. Symptoms and signs are those of a severe third degree burn. There is usually complete analgesia to touch with subsequent blistering and peeling with death of thick layers of skin. During thawing, reactive hyperaemia occurs; there is redness over the whole limb with pain, tenderness, paraesthesiae, blistering and oedema. The limb remains hypersensitive to cold for months and this sensitivity may persist for years. On re-warming there is vasodilatation and widespread extravasation of fluid through the capillary walls because of increased permeability.

The condition is worse if the patient already has occlusive arterial disease, which may be the real cause in cases where gangrene occurs after exposure to subnormal, but not too severe, temperatures; i.e. it is not really due to frostbite at all. If frostbite is present, therefore, the patient should always be examined for signs of pre-existing arterial disease which will considerably worsen the prognosis, making early treatment even more imperative.

Treatment

The wearing of suitable protective footwear and gloves is essential in sub-zero temperatures. In such conditions one should keep warm and active. Care of the feet is important. Scrupulous cleanliness should be observed, and rubbing with Lanolin, prevention of trauma and care of cracks, sores etc. should be meticulous. As soon as possible the affected part should be warmed to body temperature, but not higher. Rapid thawing is now known to be advantageous in saving tissue (a warm bath at 40–42°C for a few minutes). Antibiotics, intravenous papaverine and anti-coagulants may all be helpful. Sympathetic block or even sympathectomy is indicated if recovery is unduly delayed. Eventual gangrene can be quite superficial and the dead tissues separate spontaneously.

PAINFUL CONDITIONS OF VENOUS ORIGIN

Pain which is venous in origin may arise due to:

1. Venous incompetence.
2. Inflammatory conditions.

Venous incompetence

Superficial varicosity is extremely common in white Western populations but rare in Oriental countries. It is also rare in pure-blooded Negroes but common in populations of mixed blood. There is a definite family trait and females are more commonly affected than males in the ratio of 10 to 1.

The condition often commences with pregnancy, usually the first but it may not present until after the second. It is commonly bilateral. The involved vein may be of the long or short saphenous system, of the superficial communicating veins, or of the deep perforating veins. The vein is lengthened, tortuous and thickened.

Incompetence is caused by failure of the venous cusps to close when the superficial venous pressure rises. This may be due to atrophy or rupture of the cusp or dilatation of the valve ring with increasing venous back pressure at the periphery. There is evidence to suggest that the basic lesion is in the vein wall rather than in the valve. Increasing fibrosis in the vein wall is found involving the muscle and collagen layers.

The patient complains of chronic aching pain in the calf and foot, aggravated by prolonged standing and immediately relieved by rest or elevation of the leg. The patient may also complain of night cramps in the foot or calf which are sometimes quite severe. Relief is often obtained by repeatedly moving the legs from one position to another – the so-called 'restless leg syndrome'. This syndrome may occur without any obvious superficial varicosities and may be due to a localized deep venous incompetence.

Treatment

Relief of pain is obtained by treatment of the varicosities by surgery or by sclerotherapy. The latter is indicated where the varicose bunches are localized, where there is no incompetence at the origin of the long or short saphenous vein or when the patient is unfit for surgery. Localized phlebitis or periphlebitis may make removal impossible and sclerotherapy is also indicated here.

The provision of elasticated support hose or supporting bandages will provide temporary relief. In cases where the main complaint is of 'heavy legs', 'restless legs' and 'night cramps' a two month course of dihydroxyethylrutoside (250 mg × 3 to 4 times daily) should be given and repeated after a further two month interval.

Deep venous incompetence

This is usually a late sequel of deep thrombophlebitis but in rare cases it is congenital.

The deep vein is occluded by thrombosis during the acute episode and after a period of time varying from weeks to months the occlusion gives way to incompetence as the vein is recanalized. Rarely the deep vein remains occluded. Normally as the valves are involved in the retracting organized thrombus, they are rendered incompetent and this produces deep venous back pressure with swelling of the calf and ankle accompanied by chronic aching pain relieved by rest and elevation.

Long-standing deep venous back-pressure may produce a post-thrombotic ulcer at the malleolar level. This is usually preceded by a slowly developing area of subcutaneous, tender, painful induration with pigmentation of the overlying skin.

Deep vein thrombosis is best treated conservatively by control of the swelling with firm bandaging, the use of diuretics, sleeping with the foot of the bed elevated by an optimum 20 cm and calf muscle and ankle exercises to improve the venous return. In the semi-acute stage treatment with indomethacin will give rapid improvement but in the low grade chronic variety where an indolent, cyanosed, indurated patch surrounded by cellulitis develops treatment is often prolonged.

The condition may respond to stanozolol (5 mg twice daily) in repeated two week courses with a seven to ten day rest period between each course. Early institution of this regime following an episode of deep phlebitis will avert many of the late sequelae.

Local treatment with a heparin cream such as Heparinoid or Butazolidine cream is sometimes most effective.

a. Night cramps

These usually respond to quinine sulphate 500–1000 mg at night before retiring, for a period of 7–10 days with a similar period free of treatment before another course is given to prevent any cumulative effect.

b. 'The restless leg syndrome'

This often responds to dihydroxyethylruteside (see above) given for a two month period and repeated at two monthly intervals, for long periods.

c. Chronic post-thrombotic pain

This will benefit from a combination of moderate elevation at rest and support by firm bandaging or wearing supporting stockings where appropriate. All bandaging in the chronic postphlebitis limb should be double, the first layer being applied from the toes to just below or above the knee depending on the upper level of the lesion, and the second from the ankle upwards to cover the first. These bandages must be re-applied once or twice during the day if they should become loose. This regime presents the most effective method of controlling the swelling.

Preparations for treatment of ischaemic pain and gangrene

| **Eusol:** | Chlorinated lime | 1.25 g |
| | Boric acid | 1.25 g |

Calc. hydrochloride   1.25 g
Water to 100 ml

Contains approx 0.3% weight/volume of available chlorine.

The formula of glycerine and urea peroxidase:

8-hydroxyquinoline base   1 g
Urea hydrogen peroxide   40 g
Anhydrous glycerine   950 g

Intra-arterial perfusion

1 litre of low molecular weight Dextran (Dextran 70)

160 mg of thymoxamine hydrochloride

1000 units of heparin per litre

The solution is perfused into the artery by a Teflon catheter at the rate of 1 litre every 16 hours given continuously for a minimum period of 48 hours. It can be continued for up to 5 days or longer, if necessary.

Recommended Reading

1. Eastcott, H.H.G. (1973). *Arterial Surgery*, 2nd Edn. (London: Pitman Medical)
2. Haimovici, H. (1984). *Vascular Surgery: Principles and Techniques*, 2nd revised Edn. (New York: Appleton Century, Crofts)

10

Visceral Disease

Michael Cousins

Introduction

The symptoms from a visceral disorder are often more difficult to
elucidate than those of somatic origin. There are a number of causative
mechanisms and different clinical presentations, which may be expressed as vague symptoms, such as nausea, headache, fatigue, indigestion,
belching, dry mouth and blurring of vision. The clinical picture will
be coloured by previous experience, family, ethnic, cultural, religious
and other factors. In particular it should be noted that many patients,
who come to their doctor with visceral pain, are anxious or under
stress and are uncertain about what is going on inside them. A psychosomatic origin must always be considered, because an entirely physical
approach to the problem is likely to be unsuccessful.

MECHANISMS AND CLINICAL FEATURES OF VISCERAL PAIN

Pain in visceral organs may be initiated by a wide variety of
pathophysiological mechanisms such as ischaemia, inflammation or
obstruction of hollow organs. The pain can be either constant or
intermittent in nature. In general ischaemia and inflammation usually
provoke a constant pain (e.g. myocardial infarction, embolus in a
mesenteric artery and cholecystitis). Obstruction in a hollow organ,
where the intraluminal pressure rises and falls, usually causes intermittent pain (e.g. obstructive ileus).

1. *Autonomic and somatic afferent convergence*

Sympathetic and somatic cutaneous afferent pathways probably converge onto the spinal cord (Figure 1). Visceral noxious impulses are transmitted from a wide area, equivalent to about a quarter of the body surface, and yet visceral afferents account for only 10% of the fibres in the dorsal root. They branch extensively before terminating in the spinal cord and there is considerable overlap in the fields of adjacent dorsal and ventral nerve roots. The pattern of stimulation

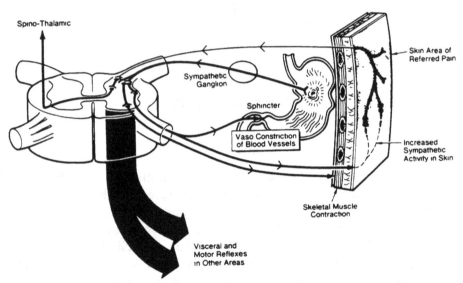

Figure 1 Mechanisms of visceral pain: 'Convergence' of visceral and somatic afferents and 'projection' to brain.

Visceral sympathetic afferents converge on the same dorsal horn neuron as somatic nociceptive afferents. Visceral noxious stimuli are then conveyed, together with somatic noxious stimuli via the spinothalamic/spino-reticular tract to the brain. Note the following:

1. 'Referred' pain is 'felt' in the cutaneous area corresponding to the dorsal horn neurons upon which visceral afferents converge.
2. Reflex somatic motor activity results in muscle spasm which may stimulate parietal peritoneum causing *somatic* noxious input to dorsal horn.
3. Reflex sympathetic efferent activity may result in spasm of sphincters of viscera over a wide area.
4. Reflex sympathetic efferent activity may result in visceral ischaemia, and further noxious stimulation. Also, visceral nociceptors may be sensitized by noradrenaline release and microcirculatory changes.
5. Increased sympathetic activity may influence *cutaneous* nociceptors and this may be at least partly responsible for 'hyperalgesia'.

Reproduced with permission from Cousins, M.J. and Phillips, G.D. (1985) *Acute Pain Management*, In *Clinics in Critical Care Medicine* Series (Edinburgh: Churchill Livingstone) and the wide convergence account for the characteristic dullness, poor localization and referral of visceral pain to the body surface. Deep musculo-skeletal and visceral pain have many features in common which are entirely different to those of superficial somatic pain (Table 1).

Visceral pain: This is dull, poorly localized pain and appears to be coming from deep inside the body. It is often close to the midline and is described as heaviness, pressure, tightness or squeezing, accompanied by nausea, vomiting or sweating. Often there is marked evidence of anxiety, which may be the result of increased autonomic activity. On the other hand anxiety may express itself as visceral pain. Cutaneous and deep hyperaesthesia may develop at a later stage.

Referred pain: Pain of visceral origin is referred to the body surface by the convergence of sympathetic and somatic afferents already described. It is usually of an aching quality, similar to muscular pain, and is poorly localized. It may be accompanied by deep, visceral pain.

Hyperalgesia: Cutaneous hyperalgesia means increased sensitivity to minor noxious stimuli. Similarly deep hyperalgesia is pain in muscles in response to light pressure. The areas of hyperalgesia and referred pain are usually quite similar and some of these are illustrated in Figure 2. However, these areas are only approximate guides, because there is considerable variation and overlap in the pattern of distribution.

Table 1 'Visceral' pain compared to 'somatic' pain

	Somatic	*Visceral*
Site	Well localized	Poorly localized
Radiation	May follow distribution of somatic nerve	Diffuse
Character	Sharp and definite	Dull and vague (may be colicky, cramping, squeezing etc.)
Relation to stimulus	'Hurts where the stimulus is' associated with external factors	May be 'referred' to another area. Associated with internal factors
Time relations	Often constant (sometimes periodic)	Often periodic and builds to peaks (sometimes constant)
Associated symptoms	Nausea usually only with 'deep' somatic pain due to bone involvement	Often nausea, vomiting, 'sickening' feeling

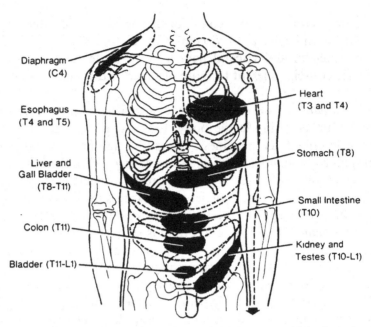

Figure 2 'Viscerotomes'. Approximate superficial areas to which visceral pain is referred and related dermatomes. Note that these regions are similar to the area of skin hyperalgesia that may be associated with pain in each viscus. The 'related dermatomes' also correspond to the spinal cord segments where visceral nociceptor afferents from each organ are thought to terminate. However there is considerable overlap among various organs. The spinal segments receiving the visceral afferents from each organ are given in parentheses.
Reproduced with permission from Cousins, M.J. and Bridenbaugh, P.O. (1987) *Neural Blockade in Clinical Anesthesia and Pain Management.* 2nd Edn. (Philadelphia: J.B. Lippincott)

2. Reflex neural activity

Visceral pain is often associated with muscle spasm and reflexes in other organs, such as duodenal spasm following severe gastric irritation. Again this is explained by convergence of visceral afferents. An example of this phenomenon is the muscle spasm, burning pain and other classic signs of sympathetic overactivity developing in an arm of a patient with myocardial ischaemia.

3. *Somato-visceral reflexes*

Visceral pain is sometimes referred to the surface and equally, sensitivity in the skin may be interpreted as visceral pain. This interrelation between the skin and visceral structures is sometimes expressed as sensory loss or hyperaesthesia in the relevant dermatome.

4. *Persistent visceral pain without apparent cause*

Persistent visceral pain without an apparent cause may be explained as part of a chain of events in a self-perpetuating vicious circle (Figure 1). Another possible explanation is reactivation of memory traces following a previous unpleasant experience. This is illustrated by the patient with recurrence of pain in the arm which occurred originally after myocardial infarction.

5. *Insensitivity of some viscera*

Parenchymatous organs, like the liver, kidney and spleen, are reputedly insensitive to noxious stimulation and pain emanates only from stretching or inflammation of the peritoneum. Similarly pain arises not from cutting but only from torsion or ischaemia of the ovary.

6. *Stimulation of specific visceral nociceptors*

The common sites and proposed causes of some forms of visceral pain are shown in Table 3 even though there is often no direct evidence of disorder. Activation of nociceptors may give rise to pain. Myocardial receptors respond to chemical substances released by ischaemia, while those in the lung are activated by congestion, micro-embolism and atelectasis. Stretching of the parietal pleura due to a pneumothorax also stimulates receptors in the chest wall. Gastro-intestinal nociceptors are distributed along vessels in the mesentery and walls of viscera. They are connected to afferent fibres in the sympathetic nerves and are involved in the pain of smooth muscle contraction due, for example, to obstruction of a hollow viscus. Other sources are mechanical or chemical irritation of inflamed mucosa, stretching visceral capsule due to distension of visceral tissue and direct infiltration or compression of peripheral branches of the coeliac plexus. Pain emanating from the alimentary tract may eventually include somatic afferents, if the disease spreads to the parietal peritoneum, abdominal wall or the under-surface of the diaphragm. Non-specific receptors may be responsible for dull, aching, ill-defined visceral pain in contrast to sharper, burning sensation arising from more specific sites, such as biliary or urinary distension. Testicular visceral nociceptors behave in a similar way to those in the skin. They are located close to the tunica vaginalis and respond to mechanical, thermal or chemical stimuli.

Diagnosis of visceral pain syndromes

Careful history and physical examination are essential for the diagnosis of the cause of visceral pain. Of particular importance are:

1. *Onset.* A rapid onset suggests mechanisms such as rupture of an organ or arterial occlusion due to embolus. More gradual onset suggests for example inflammation.
2. *Time-relations after onset.* Is the pain gradually increasing or decreasing?
3. *Characteristics of pain.* Is the pain constant (e.g. ischaemia, inflammation) or intermittent (e.g. periodically raised pressure in hollow organs)?
4. *Intensity of pain.*
5. *Site and radiation,* outlining patterns of distribution due to deep visceral or referred pain. Is the site constant or changing?
6. *Special characteristics* of pain such as relation to food and relieving factors.
7. *Symptoms associated with the pain* – e.g. dysphagia, breathlessness, tachycardia, cough, haemoptysis, flatulence, distension, nausea, vomiting, increased bowel sounds, salivation, regurgitation, sweating, change in bowel habits, bloody stools, disordered micturition, dysmenorrhoea and vaginal discharge.

Thoracic visceral pain

Pain may be referred over a wide area; for example apical lung involvement activates somatic afferents in the brachial plexus (C5-T1) resulting in shoulder and arm pain, and diaphragmatic involvement gives rise to shoulder pain via branches of the phrenic nerve (C3-4). On the other hand pain emanating from the chest wall is transmitted by the intercostal nerves and fairly well localized.

Angina pectoris

The pain of angina pectoris is characteristically initiated by physical exertion or psychological stress and relieved by rest or administration of nitroglycerine. It is often transient, 'crushing' and diffuse, predominantly in the retrosternal region. Pain may radiate into the left arm and hand or to the side of the neck, into the jaw or downwards into the back or epigastrium. It is transmitted by convergence of cervical or thoracic afferents and branches of the brachial plexus. Transient ST changes may be noticed on the ECG and subsequently there should be no evidence of myocardial infarction or abnormal levels of cardiac enzymes. Many patients become very anxious at the prospect of cardiac infarction and a vicious circle of pain with anxiety develops, with severe limitation of physical activity.

Myocardial infarction pain

This is usually more longstanding than episodes of angina pectoris; it is relieved by morphine and is associated with marked changes in the ECG and enzyme levels but occasionally it is painless. *Thoracic aortic aneurysm* gives rise to pain which is severe, longlasting and radiates to the midscapular region.

Reflux oesophagitis

Typical features of this condition are retrosternal pain on bending, lying down or after eating or drinking very hot or cold fluids. Heartburn occurs in 80–90% of the patients. Oesophagitis with non-malignant ulceration is confirmed by oesophagoscopy. Treatment is mainly conservative. The first step of the therapy includes:

1. Weight reduction in fat patients,

2. Avoidance of fat, large or night meals,

3. Stop smoking and consumption of alcohol and

4. Elevation of the head of the bed.

Drug treatment includes antacids or alginic acid in mild cases. More severe oesophagitis is treated with H2-receptor blockers (cimetidine or ranitidine). Occasionally surgery is needed if these measures are not effective.

Abdominal visceral pain

Pain from the abdominal viscera is transmitted by autonomic nerve fibres to the coeliac plexus and from there by the splanchnic nerves to the spinal cord in segments T5-T12/L1. The somatic intercostal and phrenic nerves are concerned principally in referred pain but may be involved more directly if the disease process spreads to them. In a few cases sympathetic block may be helpful in establishing the diagnosis (see Chapter 13).

Table 2   Causes of chronic abdominal 'visceral pain'

Gastro-intestinal
Gastric ulcer (X-ray negative); Post-bulbar duodenal ulcer unrevealed by X-ray; Gall-stones (not demonstrated radiologically); Enterospasm; Habitual purgation; Subacute recurrent appendicitis; Meckel's diverticulum; Caecal diverticulitis; Crohn's disease; Recurrent intussusception due to intestinal polyposis; Infestation with round worms or tapeworms; Retroperitoneal tumour; Periodic peritonitis; Pneumatosis cystoides intestinalis.

Biliary and Hepatic
Stenosis of Ampulla of Vater; Gall-stones in the common bile duct;

Urological:
Intermittent hydronephrosis; Kidney stones (not demonstrated radiologically)

Cardio-vascular
Abdominal angina; Dissecting aneurysm of aorta; Cardiac failure (liver distension)

General medical disease
Periarteritis nodosa; Haemochromatosis; Porphyria; Lead poisoning; Essential hyper-lipaemia

Nervous system
Depressive and other psychoneurotic states; Anxiety states; Abdominal migraine

Causes of 'abdominal wall' pain

Nervous system
Nipping of intercostal nerve by a loose costal cartilage; Neurofibroma of intercostal nerve; Root pressure from spondylosis or neoplasm

Musculo-skeletal
Painful scar; Xiphoidalgia; Epigastric fatty hernia; Hernia spigelli

Common causes of chronic abdominal pain

Common causes of chronic abdominal pain are listed in Table 2 and some of these conditions are described briefly here. However, it should be noted that ischaemic heart disease and oesophagitis may also present as upper abdominal pain. Diseases involving the peripheral part of the diaphragm cause pain at the lower part of the rib cage. Other characteristic pain patterns are summarized in Table 3 and Figure 2.

Biliary disease

The patient complains of pain in the right upper quadrant and epigastrium, but it may be referred to other parts of the abdomen. Intolerance of fatty foods is another feature. Severe bouts of colic, with nausea and sweating, is an indication of a stone in the common bile duct. Routine X-rays and standard cholecystograms and cholangiograms do not always show gall stones. Ultrasound and detailed radiological studies are sometimes required to confirm the presence of a common bile duct stone.

Many patients, particularly young or middle-aged women, complain of right upper quadrant abdominal pain suggestive of bile stone disease, but without demonstrable organic disease. These patients may suffer from biliary spasm without stones and may benefit from a low fat diet. Treatment in the early stages consists of a fat-free diet and relief of pain with anti-spasmodic drugs.

Pancreatic disease

The main symptom of pancreatic disease is high upper abdominal pain, radiating to the back at the level of the 1st lumbar vertebra. Characteristically this is made worse by food or alcohol. Detailed X-ray examinations, when available, may be necessary to establish the diagnosis. Estimation of the levels of digestive enzymes can be helpful in this respect. Nevertheless a laparotomy is indicated in many cases to determine the true cause of the complaint. Conservative treatment consists of a balanced diet, avoiding alcohol and fatty foods, which aggravate the condition. Pancreatic enzymes may help to reduce pain after meals and a coeliac plexus block may also be required. However surgery should be used only as a final resort.

Table 3   Sites and characteristics of abdominal visceral pain

Viscus	Usual pain site	Some characteristics
Oesophagus	Behind xiphisternum	Standing may relieve
Stomach and upper duodenum	High in epigastrium	Burning pain may be relieved by eating
Gallbladder and bile ducts	Diffuse upper abdomen Right upper quadrant, back near right scapula	Often colicky Related to eating Vomiting may relieve
Liver	Diffuse in epigastrium and right upper quadrant	May be constant dull 'sickening'
Pancreas	High in upper abdomen, left upper quadrant, left side of centre of back near L1	May be related to eating May be constant dull 'sickening'
Kidney	Loin, may radiate to groin	May be colicky
Spleen	Left upper quadrant	Dull 'burning'
Small intestine	Round umbilicus	May be cramping with short intervals
Large intestine	Below umbilicus, often across entire abdomen	May be cramping with longer intervals
Sigmoid colon	Above pubis	May be cramping

Renal pain

This is transmitted by the lumbar sympathetic nerves (T12-L1). It is dull and constant in the renal angle, below the twelfth rib lateral to the sacrospinalis muscle. Ureteric colic is intermittent and severe, passing from the loin to the groin. The pain caused by a ureteric stone is due to a persistent rise in urinary pressure above the stone. In both sexes radiation of pain to the urethra usually indicates that a stone is localized distally in the ureter. Treatment should be conservative in the first instance. Inhibitors of prostaglandin synthesis may be effective by diminishing production of urine, thereby relieving pressure above the stone, reducing muscle spasm and decreasing mucosal swelling around the stone. Fortunately most stones are passed spontaneously after increase of the fluid intake, but it may be necessary to resort to surgery if they cannot be moved in any other way.

Intestinal disease

Pain due to intestinal disease varies considerably with the type and location of the disease. If it only affects the visceral peritoneum the pain is usually dull and localized around the umbilicus (small intestine and appendix), below the umbilicus and across the abdomen (large intestine) or above pubis (sigmoid colon) (Figure 2). If the disease also affects the parietal peritoneum the pain is sharper and localized at the site of the disease. This explains why the pain of appendicitis is at first localized around the umbilicus and later, when a perforation is threatening, is felt in the right iliac fossa. Pain of intestinal diseases is often associated with nausea and vomiting. Relief is achieved not by attention to individual symptoms but by resolution of the underlying condition.

Chronic constipation

This is not uncommon. Severe discomfort, which may be dull and constant or intermittent, is felt in the left lower quadrant or diffusely across the upper abdomen. Hard faeces may be detected on palpation of the abdominal wall or on rectal examination. Chronic constipation may be the result of unsuitable diet or overuse of laxatives. It is also a feature, less commonly, of congenital megacolon or Hirschsprung's disease. Treatment consists of providing substances like bran which are rich in fibre and avoidance of irritants to the bowel in many laxatives. Surgery may be required for Hirschsprung's disease.

Irritable bowel syndrome

The irritable bowel syndrome is commonly seen in young, anxious women. Bowel actions are irregular and there may be nausea and vomiting. Pain is dull and constant, fluctuating in severity and frequently occurs in the lower abdomen. None of these symptoms are particularly characteristic but it should be noted that these patients are not ill, do not lose weight and have a good night's sleep.

On examination there may be tenderness to palpation over the colon but all investigations are usually negative. Occasionally there may be bowel spasm after a barium enema. Because there is no organic disease, repeated investigations and surgery are totally unnecessary. Patients should be advised to take a fibre-rich diet, as for chronic constipation, and painful spasms may be relieved by anticholinergic drugs such as atropine. Psychological factors are important and must be considered in detail.

Uncommon causes of abdominal pain are familial Mediterranean fever, intermittent acute porphyria and abdominal migraine. In these rare conditions the pain occurs in bouts, is spread all over the abdomen and in many ways resembles that of peritonitis.

Intrapelvic pain

This is transmitted by autonomic afferents to the pelvic and hypogastric plexuses. From here it is relayed via the sympathetic chain to the spinal cord in segments T10, 11 and 12. Treatment is aimed primarily at resolution of the underlying disorder but, if this is not practicable, it may be possible to use a chemical sympathectomy described in Chapter 13. It should be noted, however, that muscles of the bladder wall are innervated by the sacral autonomic (S2, 3, 4 and 5). The urethra has a somatic nerve supply from S2, 3 and 4.

Chronic pelvic pain is commonly due to gynaecological disorders, notably dysmenorrhoea and endometriosis. Specialist advice in this field should be sought for these conditions. Other causes of pelvic pain are urinary tract inflammation. Cystitis is not uncommon in middle-aged women and is suspected when there is frequency and pain on distension of the bladder, which is relieved on micturition. Once again specialist advice should be sought.

Recommended reading

1. Cervero, F. (1983) Mechanisms of visceral pain. In Lipton, S. and Miles, J. (eds). *Persistent Pain*, Vol. 4, pp. 1–19. (London: Grune and Stratton)
2. Cousins, M.J. and Bridenbaugh, P.O. (1983). *Neural Blockade in Clinical Anesthesia and Management of Pain*, pp. 355–404 and 616–690. (Philadelphia: J.B. Lippincott)
3. Renaer, M. (1981). *Chronic Pelvic Pain in Women*. (Heidelberg: Springer Verlag)

PART FOUR
Treatment of Chronic Pain

11

Simple Ways of Treating Pain

Mark Mehta

Based on 'Current views on non-invasive methods in pain relief' from Swerdlow, M. (ed.) *The Therapy of Pain*, 2nd Edn. 1986 (Lancaster: MTP Press)

Introduction

Pain is a complex, subjective experience and not purely a sensory phenomenon. There are many factors, notably cognitive, perceptual, emotional and socio-economic, which may be just as important as the underlying pathology in determining the extent of individual suffering. Invasive procedures, like peripheral nerve block, rhizotomy or even cordotomy, are by no means certain to relieve the pain and may result in iatrogenic complications, such as dysaesthesia and persistent numbness, which are more troublesome than the original complaint. Analgesic drugs, which are so effective in acute pain, are also unsatisfactory because long-term administration can lead to tolerance, dependence, systemic disturbances or diminished mental acuity. Not surprisingly in some cases pain therapists are resorting to non-invasive methods, which may not cure the pain but are usually simple to apply and uncomplicated. Techniques, like acupuncture, are particularly indicated when the aetiology is obscure, the diagnosis is imprecise or when specific treatment is not available. Table 1 indicates some of the conditions for which non-invasive therapy is recommended and Table 2 shows the wide range of techniques which are available to deal with them. However they must not be used empirically, without a proper attempt to investigate and diagnose the complaint, a point which will be emphasized repeatedly in this chapter.

Many of these methods are simple, inexpensive and devoid of complications, but they are slow to take effect and pain relief is seldom complete. Patients and their relatives must understand the treatment, its objectives and limitations, and persist with it long enough to give it a fair trial.

Table 1 Complex pain problems, for which non-invasive methods are recommended

I.	MUSCULOSKELETAL	1.	Persistent low back and neck pain (e.g. spondylosis, arthritis, post-laminectomy syndromes)
		2.	Myofascial (e.g. frozen shoulder)
		3.	Ankylosing spondylitis and Paget's disease
		4.	Arthritis and bony degenerative changes, causing nerve root irritation or entrapment
II.	NEUROLOGICAL	1.	Intractable headache
		2.	Oro-facial pain (e.g. atypical facial pain)
		3.	Central pain (e.g. the thalamic syndrome)
		4.	Neuralgias, especially post-herpetic
		5.	Neuritis (e.g. diabetic, alcoholic or following a neurolytic injection)
		6.	Peripheral neuropathies
		7.	Other nerve lesions (e.g. neuromas, amputation stump)
		8.	Spasticity
		9.	Neurological diseases (e.g. multiple sclerosis)
III.	AUTONOMIC		e.g. Peripheral vascular ischaemia: causalgia
IV.	INFLAMMATORY		e.g. Chronic pancreatitis
V.	PSYCHOSOMATIC DISORDERS		All treatment to be used with discretion; the advice of a psychiatrist should be sought (see Chapter 4)
VI.	PAIN OF UNKNOWN ORIGIN		

Patients with chronic pain are often impatient and expect instant success or will respond enthusiastically to a new treatment in the initial stages but will fail to maintain improvement.

Table 2 Non-invasive methods of pain treatment

I.	PERIPHERAL–PHYSICAL	Counter-irritation Vibration, percussion Local applications of heat and cold Trigger points and muscle spasm Physical therapy (e.g. massage, exercises, activity, education) Physiotherapy and occupational therapy TENS Acupuncture
II.	CENTRAL–PAIN ENDURANCE BY ACCEPTANCE AND SELF-DISCIPLINE	Cultural, religious and philosophical doctrines (e.g. yoga, transcendental meditation, zen, traditional oriental methods) Muscle relaxation Psychotherapy – patient counselling, operant conditioning, modification of learned pain behaviour

We recommend the use of simple, non-invasive methods in chronic pain before resorting to nerve blocks, surgery and other invasive techniques, which may not be more successful and carry a higher risk of troublesome complications.

Vibration and percussion

Repeated percussion with finger tip pressure or a rubber hammer is a well known treatment for a painful neuroma. The initial stages are sometimes very uncomfortable, but patients soon tolerate this and surprisingly report considerable relief for long periods afterwards. It is applied at 15 minute sessions three or four times a day. In this situation pain relief is derived more from the intense afferent stimulation than from release of endogenous opioids. A similar approach is recommended for localized muscle spasm and post-herpetic neuralgia. Pain relief is not indefinite, but the treatment can be repeated on subsequent occasions.

Local heat and cold

Cooling reduces cellular metabolism and oxygen need. It also affects histamine release, lymph production and cellular permeability leading to diminished oedema formation, which makes it particularly useful for the treatment of injuries after trauma. Vaso-constriction leads to deeper penetration of the tissues than by heat without affecting the viability of these structures. Analgesia is achieved by specific effects on the small, unmyelinated nerve fibres. Early ambulation after treatment is important to prevent the stiffness which usually develops after cooling the muscles. Very low temperatures should be avoided because they prejudice tissue survival by a critical fall in blood flow due to intense vasoconstriction. *Cryotherapy* is usually performed with cold packs, but cooling is slow and the body is able to compensate for the change in temperature. There is also a lower intensity of afferent stimulation which reduces its efficacy as an analgesic compared with ice massage. For this technique an ordinary wooden spatula is placed in a cup full of water, which is frozen in a domestic refrigerator. The ice block can then be easily applied to the affected area, but prolonged exposure over prominent surfaces should be avoided to prevent frostbite. Experience has shown that it is better to wrap the frozen spatula or cooling pack in a moist towel and limit the time in contact to 15 minutes at each session. Initially patients may experience a dull, burning sensation but this stage must be passed to obtain maximum pain relief and reduction of muscle spasm.

Cryotherapy is particularly useful for post-traumatic pain, swelling and muscle spasm and is a useful adjunct to other methods in spasticity. It is also recommended, in preference to heat, for pain relief in chronic, ischaemic ulcers and in patients with chronic low back pain. It should be noted, however, that patients with rheumatoid arthritis and those with peripheral vascular disease, like Raynaud's, and marked arterial hypertension respond poorly and for them this technique is contraindicated.

Heat is used primarily to promote analgesia, sedation and muscle relaxation and to facilitate massage and active physiotherapy. Blood flow is enhanced by vasodilatation with improvement in tissue nutrition and elimination of cellular metabolites. Superficial heat is used for patients who cannot tolerate cold and is commonly applied with hot water bottles or electrically heated pads, but a hydro collator pack is more refined and probably more effective. Treatment should be limited to periods of half an hour, three or four times a day to avoid thermal injury to the tissues. Heat treatment should be carefully monitored for patients with gross injuries and tissue destruction in a limited space, because the ensuing peripheral vasodilatation can cause an increase in swelling which is dangerous in this situation. Care is also needed when the circulation is impaired or there is diminished sensation, particularly in scars when heat is not dissipated sufficiently rapidly to avoid tissue damage.

Infra-red apparatus consists of an incandescent bulb with a reflector. Heat intensity is controlled by regulation of the distance between the source and the skin surface. The therapist is able to observe the area being treated which is an additional safeguard, unlike heating pads or a hydro collator pack. The whirlpool bath is a clumsy method of convection heating with considerable difficulties for a patient with impaired mobility who has to climb into the tank for treatment.

Ultra-sound is the only method capable of heating deep tissues and is therefore the treatment of choice for patients with arthritic joints. Only trained personnel should undertake the procedure, in which the various parameters are measured accurately. Delivery time is short, but only limited areas can be treated in any one session.

Other local therapy: This is a greatly under-rated treatment in most pain relief clinics. There are many different modalities, of which heat and cold have already been described. In addition there are also soft tissue massage and graduated exercises. The main objectives of physical therapy are restoration of function and physical activity. In many cases there is widespread stiffness or muscle weakness as a result of the chronic pain and disability is increased out of all proportion to the underlying pathology. Patients must learn to understand their disease and, as they get pain relief, be encouraged to increase the range of movements. This is particularly important in chronic back pain.

Muscle supports, such as cervical collars, spinal braces and corsets, reduce pain by limiting movement. A lumbar brace, for example, compensates for the loss of muscle tone in the abdominal wall. By supporting the viscera there is less tension on the vertebral column and corresponding improvement in the chronic back pain. However, all these supports should be used with discretion and reviewed periodically. Patients get used to them, like a walking stick, and are reluctant to do without them. This attitude not only retards progress in improving the state of musculature, but perpetuates the invalid role, which many of these individuals adopt.

Trigger points and myofascial pain

Trigger points are localized areas of focal irritation, sometimes recognized as tender nodules in the substance of a muscle or in their ligamentous attachments to bone. They are widely distributed in the back of the head and neck and the lumbar and thoracic regions. The common ones are illustrated in Figure 1. Characteristically pain is evoked locally by sharp digital pressure, insertion of a sharp needle or injection of an irritant like hypertonic saline. Sensation may also be referred to a site far removed from the source and the resulting pain is often misinterpreted with confusion in the diagnosis and the subsequent treatment.

The exact nature of these trigger zones is still not fully understood. There have been reports of fibrous tissue reaction, waxy degeneration of muscle fibres, destruction of fibrils, fatty infiltration and patchy oedema. More detailed examination reveals small aggregations of nerve fibres and clumps of platelets, usually associated with intense muscle spasm. These nodules do not change their characteristics under general anaesthesia and remain in the same state throughout life. They may be an indication of local muscle irritation or develop as a result of musculoskeletal stresses during growth. It has been suggested they may be the sites of previously unrecognized injury or an aftermath of virus and other injections.

Whatever the mechanism, trigger points are the essential features of many painful conditions, which will respond to simple treatment. Difficulties arise because the same pain masquerades under a plethora of different names. For example, interstitial myofibrositis, myalgia, muscular rheumatism and fibrositis all mean the same thing. Chest wall pain, with distinct trigger points is mistakenly regarded as angina pectoris and gives rise to unnecessary anxiety even when careful investigations have excluded all evidence of heart disease. The *pyri-*

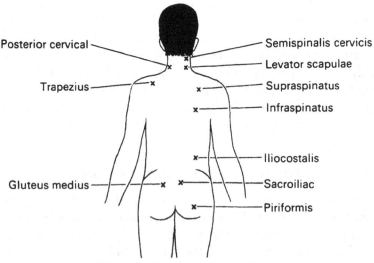

Figure 1   Common trigger points

formis syndrome is interesting in that it simulates low back pain and sciatica due to an intervertebral disc protrusion. In this syndrome, however, there are no signs of nerve root involvement or pathology in the vertebral column. The critical feature in diagnosis is pain on abduction and forced external rotation of the thigh. Similarly many forms of tension headache, whiplash injuries and obscure back and neck pain can be explained in the same way. Unilateral facial pain is sometimes due to focal irritation in the spheno-palatine ganglion. It is reproduced by the pressure over this structure by a small gauze pack inserted into the nose at the proximal end of the middle turbinate bone. Facial pain and lachrymation from this source may be misinterpreted as toothache, migraine or sinus headache.

Trigger points are detected only after an extensive and thorough search with light touch or digital pressure after rucking up the skin. Other tests include probing with a blunt instrument, like the top of a disposable pen, or injection of 0.1–0.3 ml of hypertonic saline. When a trigger point is briskly snapped with the palpating finger there is visible shortening of the appropriate muscle fibre. This is accompanied by transient pain, which makes the patient flinch and is known as the 'jump' sign.

The best treatment is local anaesthetic injection into the trigger zone followed by passive muscle stretching and graduated physiotherapy. Other methods include local freezing with ice massage or a cooling spray, acupressure or 'shiatzu' and various injection techniques. Dry needling can be sufficient, but most people prefer injections of saline or local anaesthetic with steroid.

Neuromodulation

Electric stimulation modifies pain response, partly by release of endogenous opioids and partly by recruitment of other pain inhibitory systems.

Transcutaneous electric nerve stimulation (TENS)

This method of non-invasive therapy was introduced primarily as a test for suitability of implanting an electrode over the dorsal columns in the spinal cord or over a peripheral nerve. Pain relief is not immediate or complete as it might be after, for example, a nerve block. Patients and their relatives must learn to use the apparatus sensibly, appreciate its advantages and its limitations. Electric stimulation is entirely harmless, but there are a few who find the paraesthesiae more distressing than the original complaint. Others have high expectations which are unfulfilled or accept the moderate degree of pain relief achieved, but focus entirely on what is left. Electric stimulation is contra-indicated for those with a bizarre imagination or emotional instability. Some clinicians therefore insist on a preliminary psychological assessment in addition to all the usual investigations, but this is usually impracticable. Careful diagnosis, patient selection and suitable instructions are the corner stones of this approach to pain relief. For further details of the technique see Recommended Reading.

TENS has been tried for nearly every form of chronic pain but its use, without preliminary investigations and diagnosis, is strongly deprecated. In practice TENS can be effective for neuromuscular nerve injuries, amputation stump and phantom limb pains. Brief intense bursts of electric stimulation may sometimes be effective for migraine and atypical facial neuralgia but the results are extremely variable. Poor results are obtained in those with backache due to arachnoiditis and central pain states like the thalamic syndrome.

Acupuncture

No topic in medicine has aroused so much interest and controversy in recent years as acupuncture. Unfortunately the purely medical aspects of this subject have been submerged by oriental mysticism, with cultural historical and economic overtones, allied to a strong national and religious fervour. Reasonable assessment has been difficult because many extravagant claims have been made by its protagonists on anecdotal evidence. This is no reason for cynics to decry its undoubted value and there is evidence to prove that acupuncture does produce analgesia.

Acupuncture is cheap, easily available and undoubtedly owes a great deal to distraction, mass indoctrination, hypnosis, suggestion and above all an over-riding belief by the patient that it will succeed. Analgesia is probably due to release of endogenous opioids and other biochemical changes which take place. Afferent sensory stimulation gives rise to a form of hyperstimulation analgesia (see Chapter 3). The effects are not permanent but many patients experience significant relief for several weeks afterwards.

Acupuncture is the application of stimuli through the skin surface in specific locations for the purpose of producing a local or systemic therapeutic response. The type of needle selected appears to be unimportant, because many clinicians are successful with ordinary 26 to 30 SWG hypodermic needles, but the exact site and depth of penetration are critical. Brief intense stimulation arouses characteristic heaviness and paraesthesia, a dull ache locally and occasionally referred pain. There is close correlation between trigger zones and acupuncture points, which are probably localized subcutaneous nerve plexuses and not necessarily related to Chinese meridians or recognized dermatomes.

Stimulation is achieved by needle manipulation, heat (moxibustion), or digital pressure (acupressure). It is generally accepted that the exact mode of stimulation is unimportant to success. Some clinicians even leave the needle *in situ*, once the acupuncture point is correctly identified, and do nothing further.

Pain relief is often delayed, up to half an hour, after acupuncture. The effects of acupuncture are also more long-lasting than TENS, suggesting a possible neurohormonal mechanism. Electrical stimulation can be applied via acupuncture needles. High-intensity low-frequency stimulation acts via an endorphin mechanism and is suited for chronic pain. In practice, it is often useful to start with high-frequency stimulation for immediate analgesia and follow this with low-frequency stimulation for prolonged effects.

Indiscriminate use in unsolved pain problems is strongly deprecated. Temporary pain relief may delay recognition of important underlying pathology, notably chronic inflammation for which specific treatment is available. With these reservations acupuncture is indicated for musculoskeletal pain, especially in the back and neck, migraine and various neuralgias.

Initially, six weekly treatments are recommended before taking stock of the situation and deciding if it is worthwhile continuing. Approximately 40% of those who react favourably may complain of a transient increase in pain in the first 48 hours. Usually there is gradual improvement afterwards.

Central methods

Pain is unique as a sensory phenomenon in that it is controlled primarily by the brain. Consequently the importance of mental training to subjugate the effects of physical and emotional trauma has been recognized for a long time. This is the basis of oriental cultures, such as yoga and transcendental meditation, and explains the ability of an Indian Fakir to lie on a bed of nails. In the developing countries, where finance and medical resources are very limited, there is obviously a great deal to be gained by mass indoctrination in this way, because it is inexpensive and relatively uncomplicated. The Chinese, for example, introduce this concept to children at an early age and there may be a good case, even in more affluent societies, for adopting a similar attitude. This may be particularly useful for soldiers, missionaries and other who may find themselves in situations where conventional medical help is not available.

Placebo response and pain relief through suggestion

A placebo means something to please and many non-specific methods are cursorily dismissed as of no value on this account, but of course belief in the doctor and his craft has been the basis of medical practice throughout the ages. However, a placebo has active, analgesic properties, and is effective in the treatment of headache, with a quantitative response related to dosage. Conviction and expectations of success are obviously good indications that this approach will work. Nevertheless the beneficial effects of many proven techniques like acupuncture and hypnosis owe a great deal to reinforcement by response to suggestion. This contribution should not be belittled, because emotion, social and physical components are inextricably interwoven into the pain experience.

Hypnosis and guided imagery

Hypnosis is an induced trance-like state in which suggestions are more readily accepted and acted on than is normally the case. Patients should be reassured that while hypnotized they will not be asleep, or unable to control themselves or make fools of themselves if they are in reputable hands. Nevertheless they become less critical of their environment and are influenced by ideas and suggestions put before them by the therapist. They are then better able to cope with stresses and strains imposed by a long-standing pain. Initially the subject is asked to focus his attention on a fixed object like a light bulb or, closing his eyes, to listen exclusively to the monotonous drone of the hypnotist's voice. As he becomes relaxed and drowsy the trance is deepened until he feels remote, listless and detached from his surroundings. Many patients say they feel weightless and able to float away into the distance. At this stage they are very amenable to suggestions which will make their pain complaint more bearable.

Memories, long since forgotten, may be recalled as dominant areas of the brain are uncovered. This may enable an individual to recognize fears or anxieties which have been adversely influencing his pain and enable him to put them in better perspective. Hypnosis is therefore indicated for some patients with troublesome amputation stump or phantom limb pain, and multiple sclerosis. There is considerable variation in patient response. Some readily accede to difficult or demanding proposals. Others only progress as far as deep relaxation, but the great majority respond in between these two extremes. It is this ability to enter the hypnotic state which is more important than the skill of the hypnotist. Nevertheless this is a technique only for the very experienced, because it is important to detect those for whom it is unsuitable. Some patients may develop, for example, uncontrolled panic or agitation at the recollection of an unpleasant experience and the psychological disturbance has more serious consequences than the pain.

Guided imagery is a more recent development in this field. It is less dependent on active suggestion by the therapist and does not need the deep trance-like state of hypnosis. The patient is made to relax and describes his symptoms in pictorial or symbolic form. Advisers are then able to trace important precipitating factors from past experience. Sometimes these pain images, which are a reflection of personality, give an indication of the ways in which the pain can be mastered.

Psychotherapy

Many chronic pain patients are anxious or depressed and attention to these psychological states is essential. Details are available in Chapter 4.

Biofeedback and relaxation

Continuing stress leads to tenseness and increased muscle spasm, which accentuate the chronic pain state. *Relaxation* techniques are therefore an integral part of management. Patients are instructed, in the first instance, at special classes where they learn to control body movement. They then take a more active part in their treatment, with the emphasis on self-help and continuation of the various regimes at home.

Biofeedback is a sophisticated way of recognizing and controlling the physiological effects of the underlying disturbance. With pain there are continual alterations in pulse, blood pressure and other physical parameters. Electronic devices with a visual display highlight these changes and facilitate a patient's ability to control his body functions. However this approach is no more effective, but much more expensive, than muscle relaxation. It is therefore not widely practised except in special clinics.

Religious and cultural approach

Many oriental religions and eastern cultures lay a great deal of emphasis on inner tranquillity and peace of mind. Stoicism of this kind is a protective shield against the vicissitudes of everyday living and invaluable in combating chronic pain. Meditation is a good example of this philosophy, which is gaining increased acceptance in the western world. In yoga, there are different stages of abstention, observance, posture, breath control, sense withdrawal, concentration, meditation and contemplation. When fully trained the individual is better equipped to deal with a long-standing disability like chronic pain.

Recommended reading

1. Sjölund, B. and Eriksson, M. (1985). *Relief of Pain by TENS*. (Chichester: Wiley)
2. Cho, L.S.W., Yeh, S.D.J. and Wood, D.D. (1979). *Acupuncture Manual*. (New York: Marcel Dekker)
3. Zhen, J.J.Y.J. (1964). *A Classic of Acupuncture and Moxibustion – including charts and coloured diagrams of meridians and acupuncture points.* (Kowloon, China: The Academic Press)

12

Drug Control of Pain

Tim Nash, Mark Swerdlow and Mark Mehta

Introduction

Drugs are only one means of trying to relieve chronic pain. Sometimes they are sufficient by themselves but often other methods, like nerve block or surgery, may be the principal means of pain relief and drugs play only a minor or subsidiary role. Many factors, like insomnia, fatigue, anxiety, fear, anger, depression and isolation, will magnify feelings of pain but can be modified by the use of drugs. Equally there are many ways of making a patient more comfortable, such as sleep, understanding, sympathy, diversion of unpleasant thoughts and elevation of mood which will augment the potential of any pain relieving treatment.

Currently many different categories of drugs are being used for pain relief. Some are conventional analgesics, like codeine and aspirin, with a wide range of effectiveness. Others would not normally be considered pain-relieving drugs but, in specific conditions, can produce effective and occasionally dramatic results, for example anti-convulsants in trigeminal neuralgia.

Basic principles of drug management

Analgesics are more effective when prescribed at regular intervals rather than on a 'P.R.N.' or intermittent basis. In this way unpleasant sensations do not intrude into the patient's consciousness. Each therapeutic programme must be designed to meet individual needs. An optimum level at which benefit is achieved without toxic effects, is attained only by understanding the nature of the pain, the patient's personality and the pharmaco-kinetics of the drugs concerned. For example if analgesia is achieved but not maintained, the drug should be given at shorter intervals, whereas if the dose produces only partial relief this indicates the need for increasing the dose of that drug or providing a more potent alternative. Side-effects, such as nausea or vomiting and other gastro-intestinal upsets, are not uncommon. Their occurrence can be avoided by lowering the dose or increasing the time interval between administrations. Sometimes they can be counter-acted, for example by laxatives for constipation or anti-emetics for nausea and vomiting. In general it is better to start with a small dose and the least potent drug available. Gradually these parameters are increased until a compromise is reached between full effectiveness and undesirable side-effects.

Drug combinations

A number of commercial preparations are now available comprising a fixed dose combination of two different types of drug. Their use implies that every time a dose of one is required a dose of the other is automatically taken whether or not it is necessary or indeed safe. The use of such fixed combination drugs is not recommended.

DRUGS AVAILABLE

Analgesic agents

Mild pain – Acetyl-salicyclic acid (aspirin). Paracetamol. Other non-steroidal anti-inflammatory drugs (NSAID).
Moderate pain – Weak narcotics e.g. codeine or dihydrocodeine–Combinations of NSAID and weak narcotics.

Non-steroidal anti-inflammatory drugs (NSAIDs)

These drugs relieve pain by reducing the inflammatory response to injury. They act at peripheral sites and many are also believed to be antipyretics. NSAIDs include aspirin and a number of drugs which are commonly used in rheumatology (see Chapter 8). When tissues are damaged substances like bradykinin are released. They stimulate nerve terminals directly or deform the cell membrane, leading to the breakdown of phospholipids, production of arachidonic acid and ultimately prostaglandins. Prostaglandins are important because they readily accumulate in the tissues and intensify the toxic effects of bradykinin, substance P, histamine and acetylcholine, which stimulate nociceptive nerve fibres. NSAI drugs and steroids block the production of prostaglandins and are therefore of greatest value in inflammatory pain. The former also may have a central effect, by release of endogenous opioids like enkephalin, and this action may account for relief of pain in other conditions like arthritis, musculo-skeletal injury and toothache. There is marked individual variation in response to these drugs both with regard to effectiveness and to the incidence of side effects.

Aspirin (acetyl-salicylic acid) is undoubtedly the best drug in this group, despite its well known gastro-intestinal side effects, because it is inexpensive, readily available and well absorbed after oral administration. It is an excellent, all-purpose mild analgesic agent, particularly indicated for musculo-skeletal pain. Aspirin, in tablets containing 300–500 mg, may be given every 4–6 hours to a daily maximum of 4 grams. Peptic ulceration and severe gastric bleeding, in sensitive individuals, are the most feared complications. Less marked blood loss may be unnoticed unless the stools are examined, and may be an indication of the increased bleeding time. Hypersensitivity is reflected in skin complaints, like urticaria, and bronchospasm giving rise to attacks of asthma. Great care should be exercised, when patients are also receiving anticoagulants like warfarin, phenytoin and oral antidiabetic agents. Interaction between aspirin and these drugs may lead to serious escalation in toxic effects. Consequently aspirin should not be prescribed for haemophiliacs, those with peptic ulceration or known to be on anticoagulants. It is also contraindicated in asthma, renal or hepatic disorders, and in dehydration. Its known propensity for causing gastric irritation can be limited by taking the drug only after meals and prescribing soluble preparations, like benorylate suspension 2 g in 5 ml, and slow release or enteric coated capsules. Sometimes it is better tolerated when given as a suppository.

Other anti-inflammatory agents

Naproxen (250 mg twice a day orally or as a suppository containing 500 mg) is a well known analgesic of moderate potency, frequently used in the treatment of arthritis. Gastro-intestinal complications are infrequent, but bleeding can be a serious problem. Naproxen has a high affinity for plasma protein and potentiates the effects of anticoagulants, hydantoins and some sulphonamides.

Ibuprofen: 1.2 g daily in 3 or 4 divided doses after food, increasing to 2.4 g daily, may be very useful, but this drug is unsuitable for conditions where inflammation is prominent (such as gout and ankylosing spondylitis). The onset of effect is rapid but the duration is short.

Paracetamol is a useful alternative to aspirin with less likelihood of causing gastro-intestinal problems. Although it possibly inhibits the synthesis of prostaglandins, paracetamol is almost devoid of antipyretic activity and has a less marked anti-inflammatory effect. It is frequently given in combination with aspirin or codeine. The dose is 0.5–1 g, 4–6 hourly up to a daily maximum of 4 g.

Overdosage or prolonged administration may lead to hepatotoxicity or delayed renal clearance. This may not be evident for 4–6 days, but there have been reports of serious problems after only 5 g had been given. Enzyme-inducing drugs, by increasing the production of toxic metabolites, may further lower the safety margin. Paracetamol should not be prescribed if there is hepatic or renal dysfunction and it is also contraindicated in alcoholics.

Benorylate (1.5–2 g every 8 h after meals) is a combination of the esters of aspirin and paracetamol. It is prescribed orally as a tablet or in suspension. This means that benorylate can be taken by patients who have difficulty in swallowing. However this preparation is only available in some countries and is considerably more expensive than aspirin or paracetamol, but it is generally better tolerated. Gastric irritation is reduced, but not entirely eliminated, by this preparation.

Weak narcotic analgesics

For pain of greater severity, which is inadequately relieved by the aspirin-paracetamol group, weak narcotic analgesics are extremely useful. A combination of a weak narcotic together with aspirin or paracetamol is even more effective and can be used when the weak narcotic is not enough on its own.

Codeine is an established member of this group. 30–60 mg orally every 4 h is the optimum dose but this can be increased to a maximum of 200 mg daily. Codeine has a low abuse potential but large doses tend to produce excitation rather than depression. It is also very constipating and for long term administration can be combined with a mild laxative. Codeine often potentiates the effects of hypnotics and sedatives, including alcohol, resulting in sedation, dizziness and nausea. It should therefore be used with caution for patients who are already receiving these agents, or have advanced liver disease.

Dihydrocodeine. This drug, which is chemically related to codeine, is only available in a few countries. It has similar properties to codeine but is a little more potent and shorter acting. The drug is convenient for long-term administration because there are no serious toxic effects and drug abuse or dependence are unlikely. Constipation and dizziness may be troublesome in the ambulant patient. Optimum analgesia is usually obtained with doses of 30 mg orally given every 4–6 hours. Caution is necessary for patients with respiratory disease, renal impairment and liver disease. Elderly and debilitated subjects require much smaller amounts of the drug.

Dextropopoxyphene is chemically related to methadone but is a much weaker agent with less propensity for drug habituation. The usual dose is 65 mg every 6–8 h and it is particularly indicated for troublesome musculo-skeletal pain. Overdosage or drug interaction may lead to respiratory depression, convulsions and mental confusion. It should be used with great caution if the patient has impaired renal function. Sensitive individuals may be troubled with bullous skin eruptions.

Opioids (opiates)

These are not ordinarily used for non-cancer pain, because of the grave risk of habituation and drug dependence. Furthermore there are many types of pain (e.g. deafferentation) which are not relieved by narcotics. In exceptional circumstances, when there is very severe pain which is uncontrolled in any other way, it may be justifiable to allow a potent narcotic analgesic for a short period of time until definitive therapy is achieved. Patients must be emotionally stable, appreciate fully the implications of the medication and their agreement sought after consultation with the family.

Psychotropic drugs (see also Chapter 14)

Tricyclic antidepressants

These drugs are very useful in the treatment of chronic pain where there is overt or marked depression. However in a lower dosage range they are still effective in relieving the burning pain and dysaesthesiae which occur after dorsal rhizotomy, cordotomy, thalamic pain following cerebro-vascular accidents, pain after nerve injury, post-herpetic neuralgia and post-paraplegic pain. Their routine use or long-term administration is not recommended, because of problems of habituation and serious side effects. It is usual to conduct a preliminary trial for 3–4 weeks and if there is no marked improvement administration should be stopped.

Serotonin and noradrenaline are intimately concerned in the neurotransmission of pain and the antidepressants have the ability to raise the levels of these drugs by blocking their re-uptake by the neuron (see Chapter 3). In this way they are effective in the relief of chronic pain.

Amitriptyline is the drug of choice. Details of the administration are described in Chapter 14.

Imipramine is a useful alternative to amitriptyline, with less sedative action; 25 mg orally at night is the usual dose.

Phenothiazines

The concurrent use of a phenothiazine potentiates the analgesic activity of the tricyclic antidepressants. The drugs are often used together because of this effect and also because they tend to counteract each other's undesirable side-effects. The analgesic actions of the phenothiazines are believed to take place via a generalized deafferentation effect involving the reticular activating system.

The phenothiazines have varying degrees of antipsychotic, sedative, antiemetic and extrapyramidal side-effects. These are minimized by using the smallest effective dose and combining the drug with a tricyclic antidepressant. Amitriptyline (10–15 mg) is commonly prescribed with perphenazine (2 mg). Another combination is imipramine (25 mg) with fluphenazine (1 mg) given twice a day.

Anticonvulsants

Intermittent severe lancinating pains are a predominant feature of some neuralgias. Drugs which are beneficial in this condition stabilize nerve membranes and reduce excessive neural activity. These agents are effective in a wide range of painful conditions – trigeminal and post-herpetic neuralgia, diabetic neuropathy and partial nerve damage, all of which can exhibit intermittent, shooting pain.

Carbamazepine is the drug of choice in this group. It is chemically related to the tricyclic antidepressants and this may explain its mood-elevating effect. Levels of 5-hydroxytryptamine in the brain are increased and the ability of the drug to control spasms of pain in trigeminal neuralgia has made this a diagnostic feature of the disease. Carbamazepine must be taken regularly with an initial dosage of 100 g twice daily. Thereafter small increments are made (if necessary up to 600–800 mg daily at 6–8 hourly intervals) until the symptoms are controlled; lower doses should be prescribed for elderly patients. In this way side-effects are not marked but there is a tendency for drowsiness and ataxia to occur. Gastric upsets are not uncommon but are usually tolerated by the patient after 7–10 days. Regular blood counts are advisable, because bone marrow depression and thrombocytopenia are serious complications of long-term therapy. Side-effects are particularly likely in those who have liver disease or are on anticoagulant drugs and for mothers who are breast-feeding. Carbamazepine interactions with cimetidine, dextropropoxyphene, erythromycin and isoniazid should also be anticipated. Use of the drug is contraindicated in patients with atrioventricular conduction defects and those who are receiving monoamine oxidase inhibitors.

Phenytoin is a similar anti-excitant drug, with comparable gastrointestinal and ataxic side-effects. There may also be nystagmus and diplopia. It is administered orally before meals, starting at 50 mg twice daily increasing gradually to a maximum of 100 mg three times daily. The drug should be used with caution in the presence of liver dysfunction.

Drugs for muscle spasm

Spasm of smooth or striated muscles causes pain. Striated muscle spasm can be reduced by peripherally acting drugs such as baclofen or those with a central effect such as diazepam and meprobamate. Painful reflex muscle hypertonicity is helped by centrally acting muscle relaxants.

Diazepam is a benzodiazepine which, in a dose of 2–15 mg three times a day, is the drug of choice for the management of pain due to muscle spasm, including muscle contraction headaches, which are constant, non-pulsative aches in any region of the cranium, often associated with emotional stress and frequently with tenderness in cranial musculature. This drug exerts a tranquillizing effect via the limbic system and reticular formation, but it also depresses polysynaptic reflexes in the spinal cord. Doses up to 60 mg are used for spasticity. Diazepam may affect the patient's ability to drive or operate machinery and will increase the sedative effects of alcohol. It should be used with caution in closed-angle glaucoma, respiratory disease, and in the elderly and debilitated as well as in the presence of liver and renal impairment. Drowsiness, dizziness, ataxia and occasionally confusion, dry mouth, headache, hypersensitivity reactions and respiratory depression can occur.

Haloperidol is a neuroleptic drug useful in the treatment of painful episodes associated with spasmodic contractions, as in torticollis. The dosage is 1–2 mg daily. In addition to its tranquillizing effect, it may depress noxious reflexes arising in the basal ganglia. Unfortunately, its use is limited by the high incidence of extrapyramidal symptoms and its anticholinergic and sedating effects.

Baclofen: in multiple sclerosis and other demyelinating disease and following spinal injury painful spasms may occur due to the generation of pathological reflexes in polysynaptic pathways within the spinal cord. Patients with these conditions can be given some relief by the use of baclofen which is an analogue of gamma-aminobutyric acid (a known inhibitory transmitter within the central nervous system). It will reduce muscle tone, clonus and spasm with minimal cortical depression. The starting dose is 5 mg 3 times a day, increasing gradually to a maximum of 40–60 mg daily to achieve the required therapeutic effect. It may produce nausea, vomiting, drowsiness, confusion, fatigue, muscle hypotonia and hypotension and should be used with caution in psychiatric illness, cerebrovascular disease, renal disease, epilepsy and in elderly patients.

Antispasmodics

The cause of spasms should be sought. Meanwhile mild spasm of smooth muscle can be helped by peripherally acting antispasmodics such as atropine, hyoscine and propantheline. They can produce confusion, urinary retention (especially with prostatism), tachycardia (especially atropine) with cardiac insufficiency in the elderly and will aggravate gastro-oesophageal reflux. They should be avoided in paralytic ileus and glaucoma.

Common side-effects include dry mouth with difficulty in swallowing, thirst, mydriasis with increased intraocular pressure, flushing dry skin, tachycardia and palpitations and arrhythmias. Hyoscine crosses the blood/brain barrier and particularly produces sedation.

Propantheline is the drug of choice and should be administered in a dose of 15 mg three times a day before meals and 30 mg at night.

Drugs for control of oedema

Oedema will produce an increase in pressure within the tissues that will directly cause compression of nerve fibres or mechanoreceptors. Diuretics may have a small part to play in pain relief.

Dexamethasone 4 mg twice a day is effective in reducing oedema due to trauma, thereby relieving nerve compression. The usual complications of steroid therapy must be anticipated if treatment is continued for a long time.

Steroids

Steroids are indicated primarily for pain due to inflammation and oedema. A common cause of inflammation is an acute infection, which should be treated by an appropriate antibiotic. However there are some chronic inflammatory conditions, such as temporal arteritis and polymyalgia rheumatica which can be extremely painful and steroids are indicated. Prolonged administration is not recommended because this is a potent group of drugs and an escalation of their normal, physiological activity could lead to serious problems. Mineral corticoid effects include hypertension, sodium and water retention and potassium loss with muscle weakness.

Glucocorticosteroids cause diabetes and osteoporosis, leading to vertebral collapse in the elderly. Some patients become euphoric, while on steroids, but there are others who are markedly depressed, with the risks of paranoia or even suicide. Another potential hazard is peptic ulceration with haemorrhage or perforation. Suppression of the inflammatory response may relieve pain but, on the other hand, there may be an insidious spread of the underlying active inflammation. If there is any suspicion of this happening, the drugs should be stopped. In addition the continued use of synthetic corticosteroids suppresses normal production of the hormones and the patient may be unable to cope with stress. For this reason administration of these drugs must be increased, for example, after trauma, severe illness or prior to operation. Cushing's syndrome occurs after high dosage or prolonged administration. There are many characteristic features, including the enlarged moon face, hypertension and peripheral oedema. Patients on steroids need to be under constant medical supervision and should report immediately if any of the untoward effects which have been described occur.

Prednisolone is the drug of choice. The initial dose is 10–15 mg four times a day and this is tapered to a maintenance level of 5–10 mg per day when the symptoms have subsided.

Anti-migraine drugs

The treatment of migraine commonly involves the use of one or more of the following drugs. Some have a prophylactic effect while others are used primarily when the attack has started. The patient should obviously avoid any known headache-provoking factors such as noise or bright light.

Ergotamine is a vaso-constricting drug which should be taken at the onset of an attack. The dose is 1–3 mg; a total of 10–12 mg should not be exceeded in one week. Common side-effects are nausea, vomiting, abdominal pain and muscular cramp. NSAID, given in addition to ergotamine, can provide extra relief.

Propanolol may be used prophylactically for migraine and 'cluster headaches'. It acts by blockade of beta receptors in the pineal body, which contains large stores of 5-HT outside the blood-brain barrier. Central sedation and an effect on local blood flow may also be important factors in its effectiveness. Its use is limited by its contraindications and its interactions with ergotamine. It is administered in a dose of 10 mg two or three times a day by mouth.

Drugs for pain of vascular origin

Drugs in this category are described in Chapter 9.

Hypnotics and sedatives

Hypnotics and sedatives have a dampening effect on excitation of the central nervous system and may have a subsidiary role in the treatment of pain. They are indicated for those who cannot get a good night's sleep.

Diazepam (5 mg two or three times a day) and haloperidol (1–2 mg daily) are useful drugs in this group. They achieve this effect by facilitating the release of gama-aminobutyric acid, which depresses cortical function and possibly alleviates anxiety.

Recommended reading

Williams, N. E. (1986). Current views on pharmacological management of pain. In Swerdlow, M. (ed.) *The Therapy of Pain*, 2nd Edn. (Lancaster: MTP Press).

13

Nerve Block

Mark Swerdlow and Mark Mehta

Introduction

The application of a local anaesthetic solution on or close to a nerve produces analgesia in the sensory distribution of the nerve and its branches. This effect is used for three purposes:

1. *Diagnostic* – To determine the effectiveness of nerve blockade and to judge the patient's reaction to any loss of sensation in this area.

2. *Prognostic* – To ascertain the extent and duration of analgesia and to observe if there are any unwanted sequelae, viz. abnormal sensory effects, such as paraesthesiae, dysaesthesiae, muscle weakness or more general effects such as hypotension or respiratory difficulty.

3. *Therapeutic* – Nerve blocks are not an effective means of treatment for all kinds of pain. However in some cases of chronic pain, worthwhile relief can be obtained by interrupting the pain pathway by blocking the nerve or by dividing it with radiofrequency (diathermy) current or with a knife. Nerve blocks can be repeated if successful, to prolong the duration of pain relief, which is sometimes cumulative after a series of injections. Alternatively it may be advisable to continue with a neurolytic block or other means of prolonged analgesia.

Active movements should be encouraged as soon as the affected part is pain-free. This facilitates increased power and range of mobility, relieves muscle stiffness and corrects faulty posture. It is often a tremendous boost to the patient's morale that he can conquer his disability, even if it is only for a short time.

The effects of a local anaesthetic can be prolonged by the addition of adrenaline and this fact is made use of when local anaesthesia is used for surgery. However the addition of adrenaline is not recommended in pain treatment – it will not materially increase the effectiveness of a block and absorption of adrenaline into the circulation is potentially dangerous.

Neurolytic blocks

The injection of a neurolytic agent, such as phenol or alcohol, usually results in considerably longer analgesia. However neurolytic agents should be avoided until the practitioner has had adequate experience with the use of local anaesthetics. If complications arise they will usually be short lasting with local anaesthetics, but will persist much longer and may be considerably more dangerous if a neurolytic solution was used (see Recommended Reading). Long-lasting nerve destruction can also be achieved by surgical division of the nerve or by radio-frequency (electric) current.

Principles of nerve block

Local anaesthetic solutions block the conduction of impulses in nerve fibres by interfering with the flow of Na and K ions across the nerve membrane. They are particularly effective in nerves which have only a thin myelin sheath, such as the C-fibres which convey pain sensation. The commonly used agents are lignocaine (which has a rapid onset of action and a duration of about 1 hour) and bupivacaine (which is more powerful and much longer lasting, 4–8 hours). However, after nerve block or even trigger point injection, pain relief often lasts much longer than this, partly because the pain relief produced by the block permits freer movement and this will allow removal of some algogenic metabolites. Also the nerve block may break the vicious cycle of pain → tension and muscle spasm → pain. (See Figure 3, Chapter 3 and Figure 1, Chapter 10).

Nerve blocks are better avoided in patients receiving anticoagulants, in whom deep injections through muscular tissues (e.g. paravertebral block) can cause post-injection haematoma or even large haemorrhage.

Premedication with sedative or analgesic drugs is seldom necessary before injections. They should be particularly avoided before diagnostic blocks, where the patient's co-operation and response to the injection are necessary to interpret the results. Nevertheless painful needle insertions can be very distressing and occasionally cause a reflex fall in blood pressure with faintness, pallor, nausea and vomiting. Should this occur the injection must be stopped at once, the head of the table lowered and oxygen administration and other resuscitative measures adopted as necessary.

Before performing a nerve block it is advisable to draw the pain distribution on the patient's skin with a marking pencil or pen and then refer to the dermatome chart (Figure 1) which indicates the actual innervation of the painful dermatome. Allowance must be made however for referred pain (see Chapter 3).

Injection solutions and other methods used

1. Local anaesthetics – Reversible blocks, analgesia of limited duration (e.g. lignocaine, prilocaine, bupivacaine).
2. Prolonged analgesia –
   a. Neurolytic solutions – e.g. Phenol (6–10% in water or water and glycerine).
   – Alcohol.

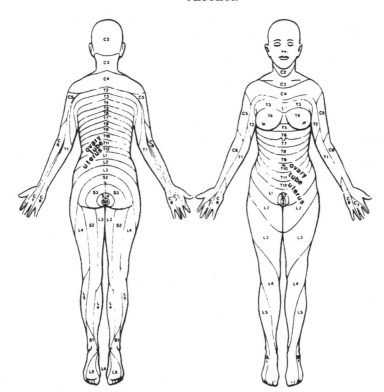

Figure 1 Dermatomal representation.

   b. Nerve destruction – surgery
                        – Heat (radio-frequency thermal lesions)
                        – Cold (cryo-analgesia)

Technique – general considerations

Many peripheral nerve blocks are simple and effective but, apart from manual dexterity in needle manipulation, the operator must be familiar with the relevant anatomy and understand the neurophysiology of pain transmission.

Simple basic rules

1.   *Explanation.* The procedure should be explained to the patient in simple terms. He should be warned in advance when the needle will be inserted, told not to move and asked to report any untoward sensation, such as burning pain or dysaesthesia, or if he experiences any muscle weakness.

2.   *Aseptic conditions* must be observed at all times. The operator should wash his hands and wear sterile gloves as for a minor operation. The site of administration is cleaned with an antiseptic, preferably coloured to make it easily distinctive from the local anaesthetic solution. Needles should be sterile, checked for patency and sharpness, short bevelled and of adequate length. They should never be inserted right up to the hub in case they break, for subsequent retrieval would be difficult. A fine rubber marker is helpful if the needle has to be advanced after striking a preliminary bony landmark (e.g. the vertebral transverse process).

3.   *Needle insertions* should be slow, gentle and deliberate, if possible after preliminary local anaesthetic infiltration of the tissues. Repeated, jerky movements are unnecessarily painful and potentially a danger to the nerve.

4.   *Correct placement of the needle tip* may be confirmed by paraesthesia in the sensory distribution of the nerve. Sometimes this is difficult to elicit, particularly if the course of the nerve is abnormal or if the tissues are distorted by oedema or fibrous tissue after previous surgery. Nerve block monitors, which provide electric stimuli by passing a very small electric current (6–8 volts, 2 Hz) along the shaft of the needle, are easy to construct and very helpful in these situations.

5.   *Preliminary aspiration,* with the aid of a syringe, is essential before injection. The presence of blood indicates entry into a blood vessel,

cerebro-spinal fluid means the tip is in the subarachnoid space, whereas air will be aspirated if the needle has punctured the pleura of the lung. Severe pain in the distribution of the nerve may mean the nerve is pierced by the needle. In all these situations the needle must be readjusted until there is no response.

6. *Monitor the patient at all times.* Nerve blocks are usually trouble-free but this should not lead to false complacency. Complications are rare, but do occur, and are serious, unless anticipated and treated as soon as they are recognized. There may be a sudden fall in blood pressure, commonly due to intravascular injection or toxic absorption after use of large volumes of local anaesthetic. Difficulty in breathing is more uncommon but is very distressing unless relieved by the inhalation of oxygen or, if necessary, by control of the ventilation. Allergic reactions are also rare but should be looked for in those who exhibit other manifestations of sensitivity, e.g. uriticaria, allergic rhinitis or asthma. The injection must be stopped immediately and appropriate measures taken to restore the circulation, maintain the blood pressure and restore ventilation. Resuscitation equipment, including the means for intubation, a supply of oxygen and essential drugs, must be instantly available. It is no use sending for them in an emergency; any delay is inexcusable and may be very dangerous.

7. *Maximum dosage.* This should be calculated on a weight basis, with a reduction in dosage for the elderly, emaciated and medically unfit and also for injections into vascular areas. For example:

Lignocaine – 3 mg/kg without adrenaline
    – 7 mg/kg with adrenaline
Prilocaine – 10 mg/kg. Seldom used with adrenaline
Bupivacaine – 2 mg/kg. Seldom used with adrenaline

Post-injection care

The patient should be kept under observation for some time after treatment before being allowed to go home. This enables complications such as hypotension, pneumothorax, muscle weakness or unexpected toxic effects to be recognized and treated appropriately. Delayed effects are particularly likely to arise when large volumes of local anaesthetic solution have been used. With regard to chemical agents, alcohol is reported to cause secondary neuritis in 15% of somatic blocks; such a neuritis may last about six weeks; it is much less common after sympathetic nerve block. Injections in the paravertebral region often leave a remnant of back pain which usually disappears

within a few days. Finally even in experienced hands, nerve blocks
(particularly chemical ones) are associated with a certain incidence of
complications, so that treatment with them should not be applied
without careful consideration.

The application of nerve blocks in pain relief

The painful conditions for which this treatment is employed can to
some extent be differentiated according to whether sympathetic or
somatic nerves are involved, although there are many conditions
where block of both types of innervation will be required before
adequate pain relief is obtained. The common and more useful nerve
blocking procedures will be described here. A more complete range
of information can be obtained from the Recommended Reading.

PAIN RELIEF BY SOMATIC NERVE BLOCKING

A. Paravertebral nerve root block

The spinal nerve roots emerge from the intervertebral foraminae and
travel laterally and caudally (see Figure 2). In the lumbar region the
cephalad end of the transverse process lies opposite the corresponding
vertebra. Lie the patient in the lumbar puncture position with the
side to be blocked upwards. Sit behind the patient within easy reach
of the injection site. After preparing and towelling the field, raise a
skin wheal with local anaesthetic opposite the selected transverse
process and about 3 cm from the mid-line. Now introduce an 8–10 cm
long 21 SWG needle with a rubber marker through the wheal at right
angles to the skin and advance it towards the transverse process until
it is (gently) struck. The rubber marker is then moved along the needle
to a position about 2–3 cm from the skin. Now withdraw the needle
a little and then redirect it forward and caudally until it bypasses the
lower border of the transverse process. Now advance the needle until
the marker is in contact with the skin when the tip of the needle
should lie in the paravertebral space. After withdrawing the plunger
to ensure that neither C.S.F. nor blood is withdrawn, 10 ml of local
anaesthetic solution should be injected. The lumbar nerves are
relatively large and the advancing needle may strike them causing pain
or paraesthesiae. Although paraesthesiae should not be deliberately
sought, this confirmation of localization is an advantage, particularly

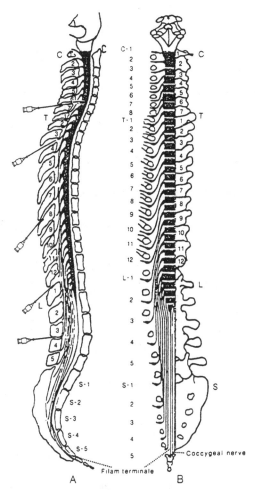

Figure 2 A = direction of needle at different levels. B = emergence of spinal nerve roots.

when a neurolytic is to be injected. Puncture of the peritoneum or viscera does not appear to be dangerous and probably occurs not infrequently, but unknowingly, in clinical practice and without mishap. In the thoracic region puncture of the pleura is an ever present risk and may result in a pneumothorax. A fine needle should be used for this procedure and advanced gently, a millimetre at a time, after the transverse process or rib has been located. A cough or sudden difficulty in breathing is an indication to stop the procedure at once.

B. Cervical nerve block

Lie the patient on his back with his face turned 45 degrees away from the side to be blocked, and the neck gently extended. The transverse processes can be palpated along the side of the neck behind the sterno-mastoid (see Figure 3). The tip of the transverse process of C2 can be felt about 1.5 cm below the tip of the mastoid process, while the transverse process of C6 lies at the level of the prominence of the cricoid cartilage. A line joining these two points will pass over the tips of the intermediate three transverse processes which lie equidistantly between C2 and C6. Raise a wheal in the skin over the tip of the transverse process corresponding to the nerve to be injected. A fine 4–6 cm long needle (21–23 SWG) is introduced through the wheal at right angles to the plane of the neck and directed slightly caudad and advanced until contact is made with the tip of the transverse process, the sulcus of which can be felt if the needle is moved a little. Care must be taken that the needle tip is not (a) in a vessel, particularly the vertebral artery, and (b) intrathecal, which latter can occur if the needle is advanced too far and passes along the transverse process and through the intervertebral foramen. When the needle is in contact with the tip of the transverse process 5 ml of local anaesthetic should be injected. Neurolytic blocks in this area are particularly hazardous. Complications include cervical sympathetic block, hoarseness (due to inadvertent blockade of the recurrent laryngeal nerve) and respiratory difficulty due to phrenic nerve block.

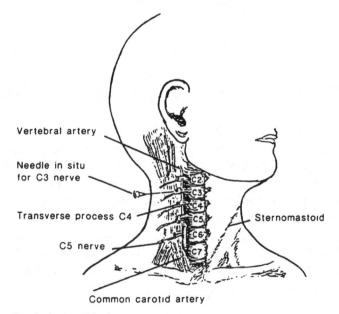

Figure 3   Cervical nerve block.

C. Intercostal nerve block

Block of the intercostal nerve is a simple, useful and, if carefully performed, safe means of providing relief in a number of different thoracic nerve pains (e.g. intercostal neuralgia). The nerve is injected in the posterior thorax just lateral to sacrospinalis muscle bulk. The intercostal nerve lies under cover of the inferior (caudal) margin of the rib between the internal and external muscles (see Figure 4a). The needle is inserted and advanced to strike the caudal edge of the relevant rib. The needle is then withdrawn a little and redirected to pass just under the lower margin of that rib (see Figure 4b) and then advanced a little into the recess below the rib margin. Deep penetration of the needle should be avoided for fear of producing a pneumothorax – a complication which is uncommon in expert hands. When the needle has been introduced in the correct position 2 to 3 ml of local anaesthetic should be injected. There is considerable overlap in the distribution of the intercostal nerves and it is usually necessary also to inject both the one below and the one above the nerve to the painful dermatome.

D. Pain in head and neck

Trigeminal neuralgia is dealt with elsewhere in this book. Individual branches of the trigeminal nerve can be injected without difficulty but this rarely provides more than transient relief. Other forms of treatment are required for this condition (see Chapter 7). Occipital neuralgia occasionally responds to repeated local anaesthetic blocks of the occipital nerve(s) (see Figure 5) as it crosses the superior nuchal

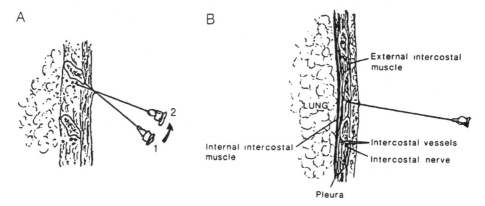

Figure 4   Intercostal nerve block.

line halfway between the mastoid process and the lateral occipital protuberance; this often needs to be supplemented with local anaesthetic block of the second and third cervical nerves.

E. Post-traumatic pain syndromes

If the pain resulting from trauma is not brought under control the pain may be perpetuated. There are a number of conditions, including some musculo-skeletal disorders, where the pain and the associated muscular spasm may be relieved by local anaesthetic blocking. Trauma to muscles and joints gives rise to spasm of surrounding muscles which adds to the painfulness; one or more infiltrations of local anaesthetic into the locality of the injury will reduce pain and break the vicious circle of spasm – pain – spasm.

F. Myofascial pain syndromes

These syndromes are characterized by pain, stiffness, muscle spasm and limitation of movement with localized sensitive areas known as 'trigger points' which are caused by a major trauma or a series of minor traumata. The condition is much commoner than most doctors realize and is usually seen in the low back and in the shoulder girdle

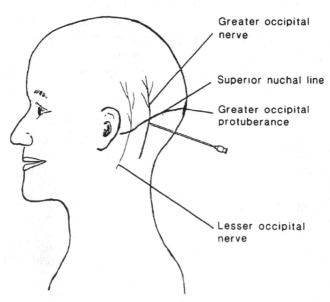

Figure 5   Occipital nerve block

areas. Injection of the trigger point(s) with local anaesthetic followed by active movement of the part can not only relieve pain but also remove muscular spasm, break the vicious circle and facilitate application of physiotherapy. Trigger points are found widely in muscles, tendons and ligaments throughout the body. Figure 6 shows the positions of the comon trigger points. These points are tender and finger pressure on them causes local and referred pain. Injection of 2–5 ml 0.25 or even 0.125% bupivacaine through a 22 gauge, 5 cm long needle can provide days of relief from pain, spasm and tenderness. In early cases one or two injections may suffice; in more chronic cases repeated injections may be necessary. Best results will be obtained if the blocks are followed by first passive and then active muscle exercises. Repeated local anaesthetic nerve blocks in muscle tears and painful old fractures relieves pain and permits mobilization which will improve circulation, disperse oedema and also reduce reflex muscle spasm and the tendency not to use the part. In *scapulohumeral capsulitis* (frozen shoulder) injection of 1% lignocaine with methyl-prednisolone into the supraspinatus tendon, the bicipital tendon and the joint capsule produces considerable improvement in the condition. The injections should be repeated at an interval of a few days and should be followed by gradual mobilization. (For techniques see Recommended Reading).

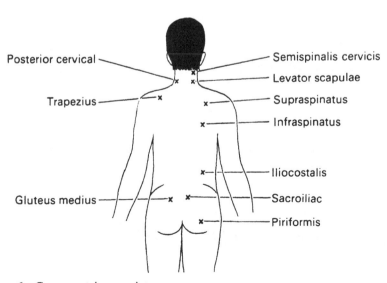

Figure 6   Common trigger points.

In cases of chronic painful shoulder, repeated suprascapular nerve blocks with bupivacaine followed by mobilization and physiotherapy can produce improvement.

G. Entrapment neuropathy

Peripheral nerves are liable to be compressed or distorted by fibrous tissue formed following operation or injury. The resulting pain is usually intermittent, but can be persistent and disabling. It is usually experienced along the line of the entrapped nerve(s) and is often exacerbated or brought on by movement (see Chapter 7). Repeated local anaesthetic block of the nerve root may be helpful. If there are associated autonomic disturbances, a sympathetic block with local anaesthetic may be necessary in addition to the somatic block. However, many of these patients are young and it is usually wiser, after performing diagnostic block and identifying the culpable nerve, to refer the patient for the possibility of surgery. In *meralgia paraesthetica* which is due to compression of the lateral femoral cutaneous nerve (Figure 7), some relief can be obtained by repeated block with 0.25% bupivacaine just below the point where the nerve enters the thigh.

A special entrapment syndrome has been described due to trapping of the terminal branch of a thoracic cutaneous nerve as it emerges

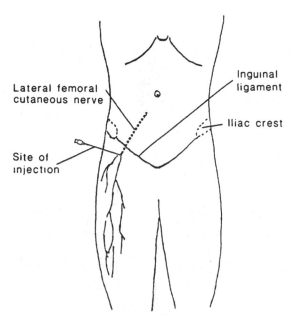

Figure 7   Lateral femoral cutaneous nerve block.

through the posterior wall of the rectus sheath (see Figure 8). The patient experiences sharp and continuous pain in the abdominal wall unaffected by rest or activity; there is no recognizable intra-abdominal pathology. The condition may continue for a long time with occasional intermissions. If the patient is made to tense his rectus abdominis muscles and finger pressure is applied along the outer border of the rectus sheath on the painful side, a small tender area will be discovered at the site of the nerve entrapment. The condition can be effectively treated by introducing a needle into the lateral part of the rectus compartment and injecting the affected nerve with 2–3 ml of local anaesthetic. Two, three or more injections may be required before prolonged pain relief is achieved.

H. Pressure neuropathies

In the elderly, in ankylosing spondylitis, in osseous tuberculosis and in cases of severe osteoarthritis, one or more nerve roots may be pressed on by osteophytes or bony excrescences at the point of emergence from the spinal canal or in the intervertebral foramen. In some cases pain occurs mostly on sudden movement, which presumably traumatizes the nerve root. The pain may respond to repeated

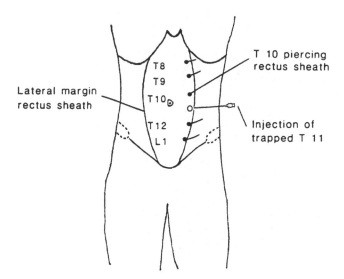

Figure 8   Rectus sheath entrapment block.

paravertebral nerve root blocks (see Figure 9) with local anaesthetic. However, it will usually be found that such a nerve block is too peripheral to be effective.

I. Coccydinia

This painful condition occurs much more commonly in women than in men. It usually follows major or repeated minor trauma to the region of the coccyx. It is thought by some to be due to trauma to the sacrococcygeal joint and by others to be due to damage to the ano-coccygeal nerves, but in many cases there is no valid explanation. Commonly the pain abates within a few months, but in a minority of patients the condition becomes intractable with considerable pain on sitting or lying in the supine position. Removal of the coccyx should be avoided if possible as it does not always remove the pain.

Good results can often be obtained by the bilateral injection of an anaesthetic solution into the last sacral nerve and the coccygeal nerve as they wind round the transverse process at the side of the upper (cephalad) part of the coccyx (see Figure 10). The patient lies on the

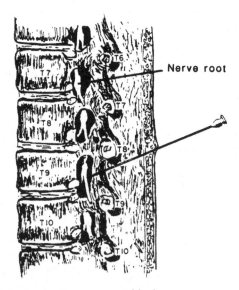

Figure 9   Paravertebral somatic nerve root block.

table in a prone position with a pillow under the hips. A skin wheal is raised about 2 cm lateral to the sacrococcygeal junction on each side. Through each wheal a 5 cm 21 SWG needle is introduced and directed medially and ventrally until it comes in contact with the lateral margin of the proximal part of the coccyx and 1.0 to 2.0 ml of solution is deposited along the edge of the proximal part of the coccyx close to its border. The first injection produces a few weeks of relief and a second, third and even fourth similar injection (each performed when the previous one is starting to wear off) may be necessary before prolonged relief (6–12 months) is achieved. Relief may be produced on one side only, in which case the other side has to be re-blocked. Occasionally also relief wears off on one side appreciably before the other side. Great care must be taken with neurolytic agents not to inject too superficially (especially in thin individuals) and not to exceed the stated dose of solution lest superficial tissue sloughing occurs. For the same reason it is important to inject a little local anaesthetic through the needle as it is being withdrawn.

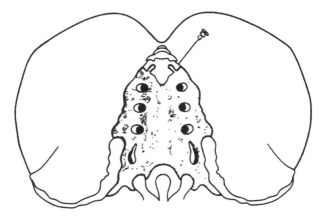

Figure 10   Coccygeal nerve block.

Extradural medication as therapy in lumbo-sciatic syndrome

Extradural injection of local anaesthetic solution or more commonly of steroid has now become a widely used method in the treatment of lumbo-sciatic syndrome and carefully employed it can be both safe and valuable. It is best considered together with bedrest, traction and postural advice as a conservative measure which might be helpful in acute and sub-acute episodes of back pain. However, before carrying out this form of treatment the cause of the pain must be properly investigated to exclude the presence of spinal tumour or other space occupying pathology. The rationale should be explained simply to the patient and the possibility of complications discussed.

The epidural injection should be given into the lumbar epidural space (see Figure 11) at about the nerve root level of the painful dermatomes. The patient lies in the lateral lumbar puncture position with the painful side downwards and is maintained in this position for 5 to 10 minutes after the injection is completed. The dose given is 80 mg (2 ml) methylprednisolone acetate suspension in 4 ml 0.5% lignocaine (the preparation should be shaken before injection). The small volume results in the steroid being localized to the desired nerve

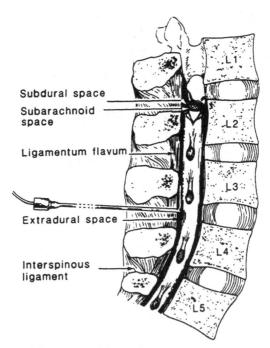

Figure 11   Lumbar epidural block.

roots. A further advantage of using such a small volume is that there is no appreciable motor or sympathetic block so that the procedure can safely be performed on an out-patient basis and the patient can be allowed to go home one hour after treatment provided accidental thecal puncture has not occurred.

Immediate but transient pain relief occurs in most patients due to the effect of the local anaesthetic. A more long lasting benefit (due to the steroid) does not usually become apparent for 2 to 3 days after the injection. Some patients are greatly helped, some get partial or temporary relief and some do not benefit at all. If the injection produces only transient improvement no further blocks are performed. If, however, improvement persists for 2 to 3 weeks and then starts to

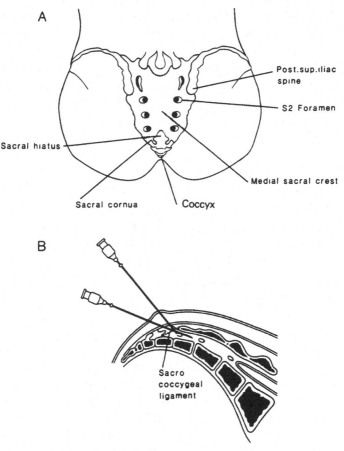

Figure 12a   Sacral hiatus (anatomical)
Figure 12b   Caudal block by piercing the sacro-coccygeal ligament.

fade, a further epidural injection should be given. Local anaesthetic-steroid combinations do not cause significant damage to neural tissues when injected extradurally.

Caudal block

For those inexperienced in performing lumbar epidural injections, the epidural space can be more easily approached via the sacral hiatus (see Figure 12a). This is situated between the easily palpable sacral cornua. The patient lies prone with a pillow under the pelvis. After skin preparation and towelling of the coccygeal area the sacral cornua are located with two fingers of the left hand. A 7.5 cm, 21 gauge short bevelled needle is inserted into the gap between the cornua and advanced at about 45° to the skin surface. A dense ligament (the sacro-coccygeal ligament) will be reached and pierced whereupon the angle of introduction should be adjusted downwards so that the needle now passes up the sacral canal (see Figure 12b), and advanced about 4 cm. The needle must not be advanced as far as S2 vertebra at which level the dural sac ends. After aspirating to make sure that neither CSF nor blood issues from the needle, 20 ml of 0.5% lignocaine or 0.25% bupivacaine plus 2 ml methylprednisolone are injected and the needle then removed.

PAIN RELIEF BY AUTONOMIC SYMPATHETIC NERVE BLOCK

Interruption of the sympathetic pathway can relieve pain of visceral or vascular origin (see Chapters 9 and 10). It may also be helpful in a number of other conditions e.g. reflex sympathetic dystrophy (algodystrophy). Crush injuries of hand or foot, in which there is no X-ray evidence of a fracture, are often accompanied by persistent pain, oedema or bruising and hypersensitivity of tissues. Continued disuse leads to osteoporosis, which is difficult to reverse with calcium or steroid therapy. This is now known to be a disorder of the autonomic nervous system, which is often unrecognized or neglected and the longer that treatment is withheld the more difficult it is to treat. Early sympathectomy (by intravenous perfusion, injection of sympathetic ganglia or surgery) is successful in many cases. Intravenous limb perfusion needs to be repeated at frequent intervals, on alternate days if possible. Improvement is facilitated by active movement or regular physiotherapy.

Other autonomic disorders – Many closely related conditions respond to sympathectomy. They include causalgia (severe burning following partial nerve damage), Sudek's atrophy and the shoulder-arm syndrome, phantom limb sensation and central pain states such as the thalamic syndrome or pain after a cerebrovascular incident, may also respond to this treatment, whereas potent analgesic drugs are seldom effective.

Sympathectomy can be achieved:

1. By performing sympathetic nerve block (see pp. 176, 179);
2. By perfusion of the limb with a ganglion blocking drug like guanethidine (see p. 181);
3. By surgical resection of the sympathetic chain and ganglia.

Sympathetic nerve block

Sympathetic nerves are poorly myelinated and they can be blocked by weak solutions (e.g. 0.5% lignocaine; 3% aqueous phenol). Pure sympathetic block does not cause hyperaesthesia or hypoaesthesia – if these occur they are due to accidental coincidental somatic block (e.g. genito-femoral nerve block after lumbar sympathetic block). Following successful sympathetic block, there is a rise in temperature

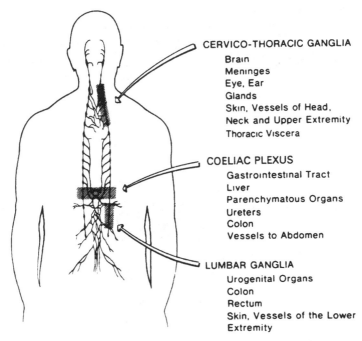

Figure 13 Autonomic nerve distribution.

of the part (subjective and objective) and an increase in arterial pulsation. Sweating is abolished in the blocked part. Clinically, successful block rapidly causes filling up of the veins of the limb. Shortly afterwards the colour of the limb improves, at least that part of it whose arterial supply is capable of responding to sympathetic block. Next the patient will report a feeling of warmth or of increased comfort in the limb if there had previously been discomfort due to ischaemia; then after a few minutes the limb will be found to be warmer than the untreated limb. As will be seen from Figure 13 the sympathetic system can be blocked at three different levels depending on the region to be treated, viz. lumbar, coeliac plexus and cervical. Each of these techniques will now be described briefly.

A. Lumbar sympathetic block

This is perhaps the most useful of all peripheral nerve blocks. The lumbar sympathetic chain runs on the antero-lateral aspect of the lumbar vertebrae; it lies in a groove between the psoas major and the sides of the vertebral bodies (Figure 14). The right sympathetic chain is overlapped by the inferior vena cava and the left by the abdominal aorta. The solution must be deposited in the correct tissue plane to obtain a successful result.

The patient is placed in the lateral position with the side to be injected upwards and the table is 'split' so as to increase the distance between the iliac crest and the costal margin. The operator sits behind the patient's back. The skin of the lumbar region is prepared and towelled. The spine of the third lumbar vertebra is identified (the iliac

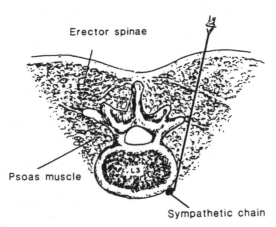

Erector spinae

Psoas muscle

L3

Sympathetic chain

Figure 14   Lumbar sympathetic block.

crest marks the level of the space between L4 and L5 spines). A wheal is raised opposite the tip of the third lumbar spine at about a hand's breadth from the mid-line. Through this wheal a 19 SWG needle 14–20 cm long is introduced and advanced forward and medially aiming at the vertebral body (see Figure 14). At this distance from the midline the needle will miss the vertebral transverse process and the first solid tissue reached will be the body of the vertebra. The bevel of the needle should face inwards. If the vertebra is not struck the needle should be partially withdrawn and then re-angulated. When correctly placed the tip of the needle will have advanced about 1 cm from the point of first contact with the vertebral body (see Figure 14); a slight forward and backward movement of the needle will elicit a characteristic feeling as it rubs against the antero-lateral surface of the vertebra and there will be no sense of resistance if air or fluid is injected. After aspiration to ensure that the tip of the needle is not in a blood vessel, 10 ml of local anaesthetic (0.25% bupivacaine or 0.5% lignocaine) are injected. If the patient is hypertensive or arterio-sclerotic, adrenaline should not be added to the solution. If a more long lasting effect is desired after successful local anaesthetic block, it can be produced by injecting 5–10 ml of 5% aqueous phenol. Two or three days should elapse before the effectiveness of the block is judged to allow the neurolytic agent to produce its maximum nerve destruction. Sympathetic block with phenol can give good results for up to six months, after which the effects usually wane.

Complications of lumbar sympathetic block

A fall in blood pressure may occur particularly in elderly patients and those with advanced vascular disease; it should be treated by tilting the patient's head down and starting an intravenous infusion. Subarachnoid puncture may result if the needle is directed too posteriorly and passes through an intervertebral foramen; in such a case the dripping of CSF from the needle would indicate the error. Chemical sympathectomy may cause neuritis due to involvement of the genito-femoral nerve as it runs in the psoas sheath; this is especially liable to occur if alcohol is used as the neurolytic agent. Pain in the back sometimes occurs and may be due to 'spilling' of alcohol in the lumbar tissues.

B. Coeliac plexus block

As explained in Chapter 10 this is used to relieve visceral pain, particularly chronic pancreatitis. Place the patient in a prone position with a pillow under the hips and give the table a 20°–30° split. The tip of the spine of the first lumbar vertebra is identified by counting up from the fourth lumbar spine and verified by counting down from the first thoracic spine. The use of an X-ray image intensifier will facilitate accurate placement of the needle.

The coeliac (splanchnic) plexus lies in the paravertebral areolar tissue (see Figure 15). A wheal is raised in the skin of the back four fingers breadth lateral to the spine of L1, making sure this is below the 12th rib; in small people and those with narrow chests the skin wheal should be made three fingers breadth from the midline. A 15–20 cm 19 SWG needle with a rubber marker is now introduced through the wheal at an angle of about 60° to the plane of the back and directed slightly cephalad; it is advanced until it strikes the side of the first lumbar vertebra. The rubber marker on the needle is manipulated until it glances off the antero-lateral edge of the vertebra and then advanced until the marker is in contact with the skin. The injection is made moving the needle to and fro a little during injection. When the needle is in the correct position there is no resistance to the injection of the solution. Ten to 15 ml of 50–70% absolute alcohol

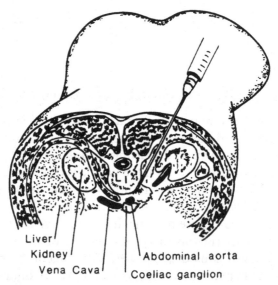

Figure 15 Coediac plexus block (anatomical).

(i.e. absolute alcohol diluted with normal saline) are injected. In order to reduce the painfulness of the procedure, the injection of the alcohol may be preceded by 2–5 ml 0.5% lignocaine. The procedure is then repeated on the opposite side.

Complications of coeliac plexus block

During the injection the patient may complain of a feeling of pain, great pressure or burning in the hypo-gastric area. This is not abnormal and he should be reassured. Not infrequently there is a marked fall in BP due to blocking of vaso-constrictor fibres. In older patients and in the arteriosclerotic there may, for some days, be a tendency to hypotension and fainting on ambulation. Other less common complications are alcohol neuritis of L1 due to accidental spillage of alcohol on this nerve root, and pneumothorax which is particularly liable to occur in long, narrowchested patients or if, due to a 'miscount', T12 is mistaken for L1.

C. Stellate ganglion block

Stellate ganglion block is useful for the relief of neuralgias and some vascular conditions affecting the head, neck and arm. The stellate ganglion consists of the inferior cervical sympathetic ganglion fused with the first thoracic sympathetic ganglion. It lies at the level of the disc space between C7 and T1 vertebrae behind the carotid sheath

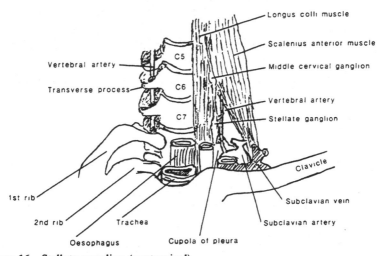

Figure 16   Stellate ganglion (anatomical)

and in front of the transverse processes (see Figure 16). Block of the ganglion usually obtunds the cervical ganglia and the upper two or three thoracic sympathetic ganglia, but occasionally thoracic paravertebral block may be needed in addition to include the upper thoracic fibres. The following is the recommended technique for block of the stellate ganglion:

With the patient lying supine and his face turned about 30° away from the side to be injected, the skin of the neck is prepared and towelled. Insert the tips of the fingers of the left hand into the gap between the trachea and the sternomastoid muscle on the side to be injected and retract the sternomastoid and carotid sheath laterally with the fingers at the level of the thyroid cartilage. The 7th cervical transverse process should now be identified; it lies about 1.5 cm caudal to the very prominent 6th cervical transverse process which is at the level of the cricoid cartilage. A 21 gauge needle 6–10 cm long is inserted and directed backwards and medially in the direction of the lateral extremity of the 7C transverse process. Injection of a little anaesthetic in the deeper subcutaneous tissues can make the procedure less unpleasant for the patient. When the needle contacts bone (i.e. the transverse process) 10 ml of 0.25% bupivacaine or of 0.5% lignocaine are injected after ensuring that the needle point is not intravascular or intrathecal. A close watch is kept on the patient's eyes for the onset of Horner's syndrome (ptosis, miosis, enophthalmos, conjunctival hyperaemia and unilateral anhydrosis of the face) which will indicate that the block has been successful. If signs of block do not become apparent within a few minutes, the needle may be in contact with the side of the body of the vertebra or it may have contacted the wrong transverse process. If accuracy is confirmed but sympathetic block still does not develop, it is worth injecting 5 ml of local anaesthetic solution near the lateral end of the 6th cervical transverse process, because the stellate ganglion is sometimes positioned there.

Complications of stellate ganglion block

Puncture of the dura sometimes occurs and should be avoided by keeping the trajectory of the needle towards the (palpated) tip of the transverse process. There is a low CSF pressure in the dural cuff surrounding the nerve root in the intervertebral foramen, so there may be no flow of CSF to warn that the dura has been punctured. Haematoma formation (due to puncture of the vertebral artery) is a nuisance but is not a danger and requires no specific treatment. Partial brachial plexus block may occur after stellate block with local anaesthetic if the needle was positioned too far laterally. It is not serious however and the patient should be reassured that the arm weakness is only transient.

A more common complication is pneumothorax due to puncture of the cupola of the pleura. It is especially liable to occur if the patient is emphysematous or if the needle is inserted too caudad. Pneumothorax is more likely to occur in tall, thin patients in whom the cupola of the pleura rises to a relatively high level above the clavicle. The patient complains of pain in the chest (accentuated by deep breathing) and of increasing respiratory difficulty. These symptoms frequently come on shortly after the block but their onset may be delayed. If the condition is progressive, the respiration will become increasingly embarrassed and there will be resonance to percussion, diminished breath sounds on auscultation and even shift of the mediastinum. An X-ray of the chest should be taken as soon as possible and if necessary repeated a few hours later. If the pneumothorax is slight the patient should be retained under observation, reassured and given a mild analgesic. With greater degrees of pneumothorax the patient will require hospitalization and insertion of an underwater drain.

D. Intravenous regional sympathetic block

This involves perfusion of the affected limb with a ganglion blocking drug like guanethidine. Guanethidine acts on the post-ganglionic neurons, first releasing noradrenaline, but subsequently preventing its re-uptake by the tissue receptors. Release of noradrenaline is painful and the patient's comfort will be improved by adding 5 ml of 0.5% prilocaine to the perfusing solution. Ten mg of guanethidine in 30 ml normal saline solution are required for the upper limb and 20 mg guanethidine in 50 ml saline solution for the lower limb.

Technique: A 23 SWG butterfly or similar indwelling needle is introduced into a vein on the dorsum of the hand or foot. (This is facilitated by making the veins more accessible by preliminary warming of the extremity with a towel soaked in hot water or a hot pack). A second needle is placed into a vein on the other, unaffected, side and can be used, if necessary, for the injection of a drug in an emergency.

The painful arm or leg is elevated for about 5 minutes to obtain venous drainage. A pad of soft material is wrapped round the proximal part of the limb and a tourniquet cuff is placed over it and inflated to 50 mmHg (arm) or 100 mmHg (leg) above the systolic pressure. This occludes the perfused limb from the general circulation, although a small amount of solution still escapes, presumably in the vessels supplying the bone underneath.

The guanethidine solution is now injected into the indwelling needle and may cause momentary pain due to initial release of noradrenaline. The affected limb will look pale and blotchy, but neither of these effects need cause concern and the patient should be reassured accordingly. Tourniquet pressure is maintained for 20–30 minutes and the apparatus observed to ensure that there are no leaks due to mechanical faults. At the end of this period the cuff is released but not removed. It should be reinflated if the blood pressure falls but this is seldom necessary; the monitoring should be continued for 2 hours after the injection. Active movements are encouraged while the patient experiences relief of pain and stiffness. He can return home later in the day.

Intravenous regional blockade often exerts a beneficial effect for 3–5 days, but needs to be repeated subsequently at appropriate intervals to maintain improvement. Although guanethidine is the most popular agent it may not be available in every hospital and reserpine 2–4 mg is a satisfactory alternative.

Recommended reading

Moore, D.C. (1986). *Regional Block*, 2nd Edn. (Springfield, Illinois: Charles C. Thomas)

Erickson, E. (1969). *Illustrated Handbook of Local Anaesthesia*. (Chicago: Year Book Medical Publishers)

Swerdlow, M. (1983). *Relief of Intractable Pain*. 3rd Edn. (Amsterdam: Elsevier Press)

14

Psychological and Psychiatric Methods in the Treatment of Pain

Harold Merskey

Introduction

Pain is identified by the International Association for the Study of Pain as

'an unpleasant sensory and emotional experience associated with actual or potential tissue damage or described in terms of such damage'.

This definition enables the physician to recognize that it is not necessary to find a lesion somewhere in order to accept that a patient is in pain. In addition even if there is an organic lesion, it may be relevant to use psychological techniques as well as physical ones in treatment.

There are marked differences in the physiological and psychological aspects of acute and chronic pain. In acute pain there is usually evidence of arousal of the sympathetic nervous system, for example tachycardia, sweating, and increased blood pressure, and these are often accompanied by a feeling of anxiety. In chronic pain, these features are much less marked and are overshadowed by different emotional changes, notably depression and accompanying widespread somatic complaints which are often out of proportion to the primary organic disturbance. Consideration of these psychological features, which are discussed more fully in Chapter 4, is essential in planning appropriate treatment.

Psychological techniques

In recent years interest has increased in the use of psychological techniques which come under the broad heading of cognitive therapy for the control of pain. For example the patient is asked to think about pain in such a way as to reduce its importance or significance. This can be done by getting him to replace unpleasant thoughts about his condition with more pleasurable ones, for example those of attractive settings or of past happy experiences. Organized or systematic auto-suggestion is another way of enabling patients to reduce pain. In this case, the patient is urged to convince himself that the pain is less troublesome by saying repeatedly that the pain in a particular part of his body does not really hurt and that it is not really pain. It may surprise the reader to know that this approach is beneficial in reducing pain. An alternative technique involves distraction of the patient's attention, for example by involvement in sport, social activities or hobbies.

It is also important to counteract the common problems of depression and hypochondriasis. Many patients with chronic pain suffer reactive depression which is secondary to the physical and social consequence of their illness. In addition to depression patients with chronic pain may also have anxiety or hysterical patterns of behaviour, associated with somatic complaints which have no recognizable physical basis (see Chapter 4). It is best to conduct a comprehensive physical examination as well as an assessment of the psychological and emotional state. The patient is more likely to accept that emotions are an important part of his problems if the somatic complaints are accepted and treated as genuine. In this way he will be reassured that his complaint is not regarded as imaginary or invented.

The first step in the assessment of a patient's mental state should be a systematic psychiatric history. For those who have access to them, screening tests of disorders may also prove helpful. They may be of a general nature or more specifically designed for assessment of anxiety and depression (see Recommended Reading). Of those pain patients with psychiatric problems a small number will be severely depressed but many more will have depressive symptoms of a lesser degree. Patients with severe depression respond well to psychotherapy but for those with anxiety and depression secondary to long established physical disability which has affected their daily lives, improvement in their emotional state will depend much more on alteration of their physical and social conditions. The role of the psychiatrist in this situation would be primarily one of giving emotional support and sometimes pharmalogical treatment without the use of more complex psychological measures. In advanced centres, a comprehensive pain treatment programme may be available to alter the behaviour of individuals who suffer chronic pain which results chiefly from psychological and social conditions (see Chapter 4). The treatment techniques used for such conditions include behaviour modification and family therapy programmes. They may apply, however, to a small group of individuals. Exercise and the withdrawal of inappropriate narcotic drugs and benzodiazepines are often important parts of these programmes. Rehabilitation often involves physiotherapy, relaxation sessions and the use of cognitive techniques described previously.

Psychotropic medication

Psychotropic drugs include antidepressants and phenothiazines for those psychiatric conditions such as depression and schizophrenia, which are sometimes associated with chronic pain. However it is not uncommon also to have patients whose pain cannot be attributed to a major psychiatric disorder. Amitriptyline is a useful analgesic in these circumstances and is prescribed in doses which are lower than those used for depression. Occasionally other tricyclic antidepressants or monoamine oxidase inhibitors are used for this purpose.

Administration schedule for amitriptyline or other tricyclic antidepressants

The use of amitriptyline or other tricyclic antidepressants is not difficult but requires care and patience and particular attention must be paid to the need to explain the nature of the medication and its effects to the patient. First, it should be recognized that the dose which is effective varies greatly from patient to patient. With amitriptyline the usual maximum dose is 150 mg (generally required only for patients who are depressed), and the minimum dose 10 mg. The patient should be instructed to take one 10 mg tablet at night two or three hours before bedtime and to increase the dose by 10 mg in each step until he obtains a good night's sleep, or indeed, sleeps slightly more than is usual. Once good sleep has been obtained, this in itself has a restorative effect and helps patients cope with pain the following day. It is advisable to see the patient within a few days of the commencement of treatment to ensure that instructions are being followed properly.

The most likely cause for discontinuation of treatment is that the patient has not observed any noticeable effect upon his pain or rejects the drug on the grounds that it causes unacceptable side-effects, the most common of which are dryness of the mouth, constipation and blurring of vision. Side-effects are usually manageable at the small doses prescribed for pain control but sometimes outweigh the benefit to the patient. Once the optimum level has been established improvement should appear within a few days, but it is important to note that a full trial of the drug requires one month's treatment.

Other psychotropic drugs

Neuroleptics are not the first choice for pain relief and their role is usually that of an adjunct to other drugs. However, they appear to have analgesic effects. This category includes chlorpromazine, pericyazine and methotrimeprazine. All these drugs have potent side-effects, especially methotrimeprazine which should be used with caution in the presence of liver dysfunction, cardiac disease and in the elderly. The patient should be given the smallest dose possible and then asked to increase it slowly to a level which gives symptom relief without troublesome side-effects. For example, in the case of chlorpromazine treatment should begin with a dose of 10 mg three times daily or 20–30 mg at night. The patient's condition must be checked within 48 hours of starting treatment because neuroleptics occasionally cause feelings of depression and may need to be withdrawn. If depressive symptoms persist after withdrawal of chlorpromazine they can be corrected by administration of an antidepressant.

Abuse of psychotropic drugs

It is common for patients to be given benzodiazepines and hypnotic drugs for excessive periods of time with the result that they become habituated to them. Both should be used for short periods and primarily to cover acute symptoms of anxiety or sleeplessness. As an alternative to benzodiazepines, a good hypnotic effect can be obtained with amitriptyline or with amitriptyline supplemented by a phenothiazine, such as methotrimeprazine.

It is seldom justifiable to prescribe narcotic analgesics for chronic non-cancer pain. If a patient has been given these drugs for a benign disorder and become dependent on them, withdrawal is necessary (see Recommended Reading).

The use of methods described in this chapter depends primarily on establishing a good relationship with the patient, based on physical as well as psychological assessment. There are a wide range of psychological measures available to help the individual and reduce his pain.

Recommended reading

Merskey, H. (1983). Psychological treatment of pain. In Swerdlow, M. (Ed.) *Relief of Intractable Pain*, 3rd Edn. (Amsterdam: Elsevier Biomedical Press)

15

The Pain Relief Clinic

Mark Swerdlow

Introduction

Ideally pain should be treated by methods directed at the cause. Unfortunately there are many situations in which the underlying mechanism cannot be identified or is incompletely understood. Nevertheless a determined effort must be made to establish the diagnosis before treatment is initiated. In this way any serious pathology (such as cancer) will not be overlooked or allowed to progress beyond a curable stage while attention was diverted to a purely symptomatic relief of pain.

Patients with chronic pain are more likely to receive the best investigation and treatment in a clinic specially designed for this purpose with a staff who are specifically interested and experienced in dealing with these complex problems.

STARTING A PAIN RELIEF CLINIC

There are a number of problems in setting up a Pain Relief Clinic; the first is for the doctor(s) to get training if possible in an established Pain Relief Centre. The method of starting a clinic will depend a great deal on the system of medicine in the country involved. In a country with a National Health Service the space, facilities and personnel will be provided by the Health Service and the doctor starting the clinic will have to persuade his colleagues in the hospital of the need to set up a clinic. As the clinic grows and demonstrates its value, it will be much easier to get agreement for additional funding.

In countries with mainly private practice and/or insurance coverage system, the setting up of a Pain Relief Clinic will involve costing considerations. When Pain Relief Clinic work is starting in such a country there may be problems in obtaining payment for treatment by insurance carriers because precedents have not been set. Many insurers are unwilling to pay for treatment for undiagnosed pain. Founders of Pain Relief Clinics should investigate local practices when planning their budget.

Specialists and family doctors in the area will have to be informed that the Pain Relief Clinic is being opened and the type of patients for whom it is intended. Obviously good results will attract more patients and unsatisfactory results will tend to deter patients.

FUNCTIONS OF A PAIN CLINIC

1. Investigation and diagnosis of the cause of the chronic pain.

2. Treatment – this is obviously the main function of the clinic. However, once the diagnosis has been established and/or the course of management decided the actual treatment can often be carried out by the family doctor.

3. Follow up facilities are important to ensure that improvement is maintained, to detect any complications resulting from treatment, to detect development of tolerance or habituation, as well as to make the clinic records complete for future knowledge.

4. Research to find out which methods of treatment are the most effective.

5. Teaching of house surgeons, family doctors and trainee pain specialists will improve the general standard of management of chronic pain.

TYPES OF PAIN RELIEF CLINIC

Unidisciplinary clinic – run by a single specialist. This type of clinic is often found in small local hospitals in the provinces. When there is easy communication with a larger Pain Relief Centre in a major city hospital, the small clinic may refer the more difficult cases to that centre for diagnosis and/or treatment. Equally the major centre may, after investigation, return the patient to the local clinic with details of recommended treatment. Any specialist starting a small **Pain Relief Clinic** alone, should from the beginning make contact with one or two colleagues in other specialities to ensure that an accurate diagnosis of the cause of the pain is made before treatment starts. These colleagues should also be consulted when treatment fails or if complications arise. A wider range of investigation and treatment can be achieved through the co-operation of a number of different specialists; this should be aimed at as soon as possible.

It is important to have adequate time to run the clinic – time to listen to the patient; time to find a diagnosis; time to try different treatments; time to follow up the case and to make sure that improvement is maintained.

The accommodation, staffing, equipment, time available and indeed knowledge may well be very limited at first and this will of course restrict both the quantity and quality of the pain relief work which can be carried out. However, a wider range of cases can be managed as the clinic grows and particularly when different types of specialists get involved in the clinic's activities.

District clinic – often at a large city hospital with two, three or more specialists involved and access to hospital facilities and beds. This type of clinic can help other specialists with diagnosis and treatment of many forms of chronic pain.

Regional Pain Relief Centre – usually in a University Hospital. Multidisciplinary and with inpatient and outpatient accommodation. Specialized skills and sophisticated equipment are available together with a wide range of diagnostic and therapeutic facilities.

ACCOMMODATION AND STAFFING

Outpatient facilities

The place in which the clinic is held will, of course, depend at first upon what is available or can be afforded. As the clinic proves its value, further space and facilities can be added. Ideally the following accommodation should be available:

1. A consulting room with table and chairs and X-ray viewing box;
2. One or more examination rooms each with examination couch and equipment cupboards;
3. One or more changing rooms;
4. An office with desk, files etc. A small reference library is invaluable (see Recommended Reading);

5. Procedure room with adjustable table, operating room light, instrument trolley, drugs, solutions and sterile pack cupboards. Facilities for treatment of toxic reactions and cardiovascular and pulmonary resuscitation.

In addition, toilet and kitchen facilities should be accessible for patients and their friends. Some of these accommodations may of course be shared with other speciality clinics.

Inpatient

Clearly an inpatient facility has the advantage of making a more intensive approach possible.

Admission to hospital may be necessary for a number of reasons. Obviously patients having invasive procedures (e.g. cordotomy, intrathecal neurolysis) will require hospitalization. Likewise patients who develop complications following outpatient nerve blocking procedures may require admission. However, admission is also helpful on occasion for diagnostic purposes and a short stay in hospital will facilitate a trial of treatment (e.g. by drugs). Sometimes admission for a day or two enables the patient to be seen by 2 or 3 different specialists more quickly than they could be seen in the outpatients.

Personnel

Medical

In addition to the specialist(s), junior hospital doctors from one or more disciplines will be required to help in the outpatients, the operating theatre and the wards.

Nurses

The number of nurses will depend on the size and activity of the clinic. At least some of the nursing staff must be permanent so that they become familiar with the organization, the drugs and methods employed, the complications that can arise and their management and so that they develop a professional approach to the patient with chronic pain.

Secretary/clerk

The efficient maintenance and filing of patients' records, X-ray laboratory reports etc. is important to the smooth running of the clinic. Adequate communication with family doctors, specialists and patients and the organization of follow-up visits are also essential features.

Co-operation should be fostered with the X-ray and physiotherapy departments, the haematology and biochemistry laboratories and the pharmacy.

Training of junior medical and nursing staff is an essential internal activity in the clinic. When a new technique is introduced the features shown in Table 1 must be explained to the staff.

Table 1

1. Rationale of technique;
2. Description of method, indications and results;
3. Apparatus involved;
4. Special nursing, physiotherapy or other after care;
5. Complications and dangers

CLINIC MANAGEMENT

A newly established Pain Relief Clinic must have a clear scheme of management as shown by the flow chart in Figure 1. Different clinics have different management systems. However, whatever system is adopted it is important that one doctor is responsible for each patient and monitors his progress. The patient should not be passed from one specialist to another without knowing who he should approach for advice or information. Of course, in a small clinic run by just one or two doctors this problem will not arise.

At the initial interview with the patient it is important to obtain a very full history of the duration, nature and severity of the pain and, if there are a number of different pains, which is the most severe and which is of somatic or autonomic origin. It is also important to note whether the patient suffers from nausea, vomiting, constipation, headache, ataxia, abnormal bowel or bladder function and whether paraesthesia, hyperaesthesia or paresis is present. Should treatment result in any of these symptoms or signs it is important that it had been noted that they were present before treatment commenced.

Care must be taken that the patient who is sent to the clinic with chronic pain does not become a chronic inhabitant of the clinic. If a patient has been under treatment by one member of the pain team for months without making any progress he should be referred to

Treatment of Chronic Pain

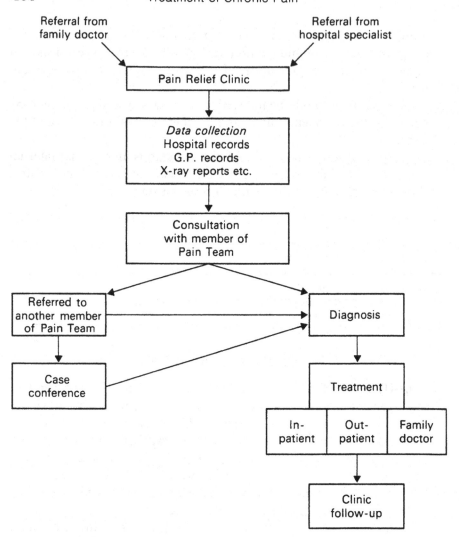

Figure 1 Pain Relief Clinic flow chart

another member of the team. The patient does not usually object to such a referral, realizing that a new perspective and approach might be successful. It is important to keep full records so that progress can be properly monitored. Sometimes the pain problem is a complicated and difficult one and none of the members of the pain team has been able to elucidate it. In such a situation a 'case conference' is held where all appropriate members of the pain team meet together with the patient to discuss the aetiology and to pool their knowledge and experience.

A small proportion of the patients referred to the clinic have considerable psychological overlay, especially patients with backache or headache; personal, social and domestic factors may tend to perpetuate their pain. Chronic pain can give rise to feelings of inadequacy, insecurity and dependence on others. Removal from work or responsibilities may be an obstacle to effective treatment.

Recommended reading

Swerdlow, M. (ed.) (1986). *The Therapy of Pain*, 2nd Edn. (Lancaster: MTP Press)

Bond, M. (1984). *Pain*. (Edinburgh: Churchill Livingstone)

Mehta, M. (1974). *Intractable Pain*. (Philadelphia: W.B. Saunders)

Lipton, S. (1979). Control of chronic pain. In *Current Topics in Anaesthesia*, Vol. II (London: Arnold)

16

The Present Status of Pain Therapy and Future Trends

Ronald Melzack and Patrick Wall

Introduction

The chapters in this book present an up-to-date analysis of chronic pain syndromes and the relative effectiveness of a variety of treatments. Generally, chronic pains tend to persist and increase in intensity unless they are properly managed. If treated early enough, some of the syndromes may even be 'nipped in the bud', thereby saving individuals from life-long misery and society from the expense of continued support of the sufferer as well as his family.

There is a need for doctors everywhere, in every country and at every level of society, to take a special interest in patients with chronic pain. Patients in chronic pain often fail to receive appropriate therapy because medical school teaching is still based on the management of acute pain. Yet we have seen in earlier chapters that chronic pain, though its causes are frequently subtle and perplexing, is so common and has such terrible repercussions that it can no longer be ignored. The cost to the sufferer may be the lost hope of ever living a normal, fulfilling life. The costs to society are enormous in terms of the economic burden of so many months or years lost from work.

Every thoughtful physician has seen patients whose pain, in intensity and duration, is out of proportion to the injury. Sometimes chronic pain occurs in the absence of any injury. Yet the physicians who know such patients personally are usually convinced that they are not malingering or conjuring up their pain for secondary gain. Such patients deserve the most careful attention. Because these pain problems are so complex and baffling, it is often important that physicians consult each other whenever necessary. In every country there is a need for specialized Pain Relief Clinics to allow concerned therapists to work together for the good of the patient and society at large. Governments must be prevailed upon to make funds available for at least a few such clinics, which are usually most effective when they are located in large cities with a medical centre. In the long run, the expenditure for such clinics is far less than the costs to society for support of people who cannot work or live productively because of unremitting suffering.

The problem of prevention

Ideas for the prevention of pain range widely in feasibility. Many working situations which inflict repeated small injuries are ignored while others have achieved a good safety record. The gnarled, scarred arthritic hands of the deep-sea fisherman on a trawler hasten the end of his active life at sea. They are unnecessarily accepted as a fact of life. In many cases of low back pain, small tears of muscle and ligaments during excessive contraction are suspected as a common cause. If true, then it is reasonable to expect that a combination of physical exercise and improved work habits could reduce this nearly universal condition with its pain and economic loss. The number of people who suffer chronic pain as a result of injury in car accidents could clearly be decreased by better car design and laws which lower the maximum speed.

War is yet another cause of frightful suffering. New weapons produce horrible injuries and, at the same time, improved medical procedures have raised the survival rate. All politicians should, on a regular basis, visit veterans' hospitals to see the gruesome nature of the injuries and the effect of the chronic suffering on those men. Perhaps such a procedure might contribute to the abolition of war and the inevitable pain and suffering it inflicts on countless people.

At a more feasible level, there are many ways to decrease the probability of suffering. Surgical incisions, tooth extractions, even episiotomies are necessary, but a proportion of them produce prolonged pain and discomfort, particularly when nerves are injured.

With study and modification of technique, many of these pains could be avoided. The more extensive the surgery the more likely the chronic pain, and yet these 'side effects' are often neglected while patient and doctor concentrate on the original reason for the operation. Hopefully, pain clinics will play a role in preventing iatrogenic pain by developing effective education programmes.

We must continue to make every effort to cure the fundamental origins of disease but it is equally important to study ways of preventing pain occurring. Painful diseases follow damage to nerves by injury, by surgeons, by infection and by poisons. We have discussed injury by accidents, war and surgery, but virus infection remains a problem. Shingles (herpes zoster) is followed in a proportion of cases by post-herpetic neuralgia – a prolonged, continuous pain of such intensity that it ruins the lives of some older people. The disease is normally short with painful virus infection of peripheral nerves. It is rational to treat the disease in its early stages because of the danger of subsequent prolonged pain.

Two common medical conditions – alcoholism and diabetes – are sometimes associated with severe pain due to the destruction of nerves. We need to understand why alcoholism and diabetes cause nerve damage in order to prevent that damage. The future, we hope, will bring an increasing recognition of all these problems as well as steps that will lead to their solution.

Prophylaxis as opposed to treatment is a much neglected area of our training. This is particularly true of low back pain which is so common. Teaching people how to lift properly and exercise their muscles is vitally important in preventing this condition. It should be carried out by people who have periodic episodes of pain as well as by people without pain because we know that a high proportion of people are certain to develop this crippling pain problem.

The need for research

The puzzle of pain, as we have seen, is far from solved. Increased research is clearly necessary. We need to know a great deal more about the incidence, underlying mechanisms and response to treatment of many pain conditions in different countries. Accurate records would facilitate information retrieval and meaningful assessment of the efficacy of new drugs together with the comparative value of different forms of treatment. Clinical research of this kind is as important as the more scientific approach in the laboratory. The number of scientists who work on the problem is small in comparison with the magnitude of its importance. We have a remarkable capacity to forget pains that we have suffered in the past, and it is often difficult to comprehend the suffering of another person. Research time and money are devoted to many problems of obvious clinical significance, but pain receives far less attention. Yet, there are few problems more worthy of human endeavour than the relief of pain and suffering.

Glossary

Allodynia   Pain due to a stimulus which does not normally provoke pain.

Analgesia   Absence of pain in response to stimulation which would normally be painful.

Anaesthesia dolorosa   Pain in an area or region which is anaesthetic.

Central pain   Pain associated with a lesion of the central nervous system.

Deafferentation   Nerve cells disconnected from normal afferent input.

Dysaesthesia   An unpleasant abnormal sensation, whether spontaneous or evoked.

Hyperaesthesia   Increased sensitivity to stimulation, excluding the special senses.

Hyperalgesia   An increased response to a stimulus which is normally painful.

Hyperpathia   A painful syndrome, characterized by increased reaction to a stimulus, especially a repetitive stimulus, as well as an increased threshold.

Hypoaesthesia   Decreased sensitivity to stimulation, excluding the special senses.

Hypoalgesia   Diminished pain in response to normally painful stimulus.

Inhibition   A restraining effect.

Lancinating   Intermittent sharp, stabbing or shooting (pain).

Neuralgia   Pain in the distribution of a nerve or nerves.

Neuritis   Inflammation of a nerve or nerves.

Neurogenic   Arising from nerves.

Neuropathy   A disturbance of function or pathological change in a nerve; in one nerve, mononeuropathy; in several nerves, mononeuropathy multiplex; if diffuse and bilateral, polyneuropathy.

Nociceptor   A receptor specifically sensitive to a noxious stimulus or to a stimulus which would become noxious if prolonged.

Noxious stimulus   A noxious stimulus is one which is damaging to normal tissues.

Pain threshold   The least experience of pain which a subject can recognize.

Pain tolerance level   The greatest level of pain which a subject is prepared to tolerate.

Paraesthesia   An abnormal sensation, whether spontaneous or evoked.

Index